T0213562

Delivering Compassionate Care

Sarah Ellen Braun • Patricia Anne Kinser

Editors

Delivering Compassionate Care

A Mindfulness Curriculum
for Interdisciplinary Healthcare
Professionals

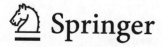 Springer

Editors
Sarah Ellen Braun
Department of Neurology
School of Medicine
Virginia Commonwealth University
Richmond, VA, USA

Patricia Anne Kinser
School of Nursing
Virginia Commonwealth University
Richmond, VA, USA

ISBN 978-3-030-91064-8   ISBN 978-3-030-91062-4   (eBook)
https://doi.org/10.1007/978-3-030-91062-4

This Springer imprint is published by the registered company Springer Nature Switzerland AG
The registered company address is: Gewerbestrasse 11, 6330 Cham, Switzerland

Contents

Part I

Introduction and Overview

How to Use This Book: Teaching and Learning Mindfulness for Healthcare Professionals

Patricia Anne Kinser and Sarah Ellen Braun

Welcome to the book *Delivering compassionate care: A mindfulness curriculum for interdisciplinary healthcare professionals.* This book is the manual to deliver an evidenced-based course for reducing stress and burnout in healthcare professionals and students. This curriculum is designed to help address burnout and improve patient-centered care by providing training in compassion and mindful attention. It is a structured skills-based manual complete with resources for full implementation and dissemination of this evidence-based course.

Each chapter in this book contains resources for applying mindfulness and compassion in the context of healthcare to reduce stress, improve well-being, and enhance patient-centered care. This manual is unique in that it can be followed in a linear fashion or can be used modularly to suit the needs of specific settings. The curriculum contains didactic content and specific examples of practices; hence, it is easily adaptable for use by groups and classes of various sizes and structure. This curriculum is intended for all disciplines of healthcare professionals and students. This book can be used in two ways: as a textbook for a course (for example, there is didactic content and examples of practices in which the student can engage) or as an instructor manual for those wishing to teach the curriculum (for example, there is material for each chapter containing "tips for instructors").

The editors of this book, Drs. Sarah Ellen Braun and Patricia Anne Kinser, developed this curriculum originally as an interprofessional education course at Virginia Commonwealth University. We also adapted the course to facilitate offerings within specific departments: e.g., Mindfulness Training for Critical Care Fellows and

P. A. Kinser
School of Nursing, Virginia Commonwealth University, Richmond, VA, USA
e-mail: kinserpa@vcu.edu

S. E. Braun (✉)
Department of Neurology, School of Medicine, Virginia Commonwealth University, Richmond, VA, USA
e-mail: sarah.braun@vcuhealth.org

Mindfulness and Compassion for Training Psychotherapists. We have conducted several research studies with findings to support the use of this curriculum to prevent and treat burnout in interdisciplinary healthcare professionals. Results of these studies demonstrate the curriculum's feasibility and acceptability in healthcare professionals and students as well as efficacy in stress and burnout reduction with increases in dispositional mindfulness.

We developed this curriculum because we identified gaps existing in other mindfulness-based interventions and found minimal resources for educating and disseminating this information to healthcare professionals. This manual is intended to fill these gaps and offer a novel, evidenced-based, interdisciplinary course for healthcare professionals. To our knowledge, this is the only evidence-based workbook and resource guide that provides a mindfulness and compassion curriculum tailored specifically to the life and work of interdisciplinary healthcare professionals and students (rather than other books, which focus on how healthcare professionals should teach mindfulness to patients). We are pleased to share this curriculum with you, so that you may implement this in clinical and/or academic settings.

This book is separated into two parts. Part I is the Introduction and Overview, whereby Chaps. 2, 3, and 4 provide background information that is critical to understanding the key concepts of mindfulness and how it is important for healthcare professionals. Part II is the Curriculum, made up of eight modules. These modules are organized by (a) key concepts, (b) suggested activities and practices for each session, (c) tips for instructors, (d) resources, and (e) formal mindful movement and meditation practice. For those who will be facilitating this curriculum, we recommend making the most of your setting by engaging transdisciplinary experts to contribute to the implementation of the course. For example, you might invite clinicians who practice mindfulness to engage in discussions with the participants. As another example, you might invite local yoga or meditation teachers to lead the mindfulness practices, if you do not have experience in leading those aspects of the curriculum.

For those who will be leading the curriculum: We would like to remind you that the most important active ingredient of the curriculum is the development of one's personal mindfulness practice, including that of the instructor teaching the course. We recommend that any instructors of this curriculum have a consistent mindfulness or contemplative practice. It is almost impossible to lead the activities and discussions in this curriculum without a thorough personal understanding of the challenges and benefits of maintaining a consistent mindfulness practice. The foundational aspects of mindfulness, such as nonjudgmental attention to the present moment, will be critical for being able to attend to participants' comments and to support them in their mindful journey.

This manual introduces an evidenced-based mindfulness and compassion curriculum to improve well-being and promote flourishing for healthcare professionals. This suggests that by training individual-level mindfulness and compassion, we can improve healthcare well-being. Nevertheless, the current burnout crisis in healthcare is not an individual-level problem but rather a system-level one. If we do not work to change our systems, then we cannot hope to truly address the needs of our healthcare professionals. These system-level changes require a drastic re-prior-itization of the patient-provider relationship over money. Thus, this manual should be interpreted and delivered with the understanding that compassionate patient care requires both individual- and system-level responsibilities. Our hope is that with increasing attention on healthcare professional well-being, patient-centered care, and the overall functioning of healthcare, we can shift the tides to prioritize these topics over and above the for-profit business model of our current healthcare system.

Patricia Anne Kinser Ph.D., WHNP-BC, RN, FAAN, is a tenured professor, nurse scientist, and nurse practitioner at the Virginia Commonwealth University School of Nursing. Dr. Kinser's program of research is focused on two areas: first, she studies mindfulness interventions to enhance resilience-building in interdisci-plinary healthcare professionals, with the long-term goal to improve patient care quality and safety; second, she explores biobehavioral mechanisms underlying depression and she develops and tests innovative non-pharmacologic symptom management strategies. Her interdisciplinary research studies have been funded by sources such as the National Institutes of Health, the American Nurses Foundation, and Sigma Theta Tau International. Dr. Kinser is a Governor-Appointee to the Virginia Board of Health, a practicing board-certified Women's Health Nurse Practitioner, and a Fellow in the American Academy of Nursing.

Sarah Ellen Braun PhD, LCP, is a licensed clinical psychologist and neuropsy-chology fellow completing her fellowship training at Virginia Commonwealth University in the Division of Neuro-Oncology. She completed her Ph.D. in clinical psychology at Virginia Commonwealth University where she co-developed the intervention Mindfulness for Interdisciplinary Healthcare Professionals (MIHP). At VCU, she taught the course to more than 100 faculty, staff, residents, and students across disciplines. Much of Dr. Braun's research has focused on mindfulness train-ing for healthcare professionals. She is the author of several peer-reviewed papers and book chapters, including a recent paper demonstrating the effectiveness of MIHP in reducing burnout, stress, and daily activity impairment. She received the 2019 Elizabeth Fries Scholarship in Cancer Prevention and Control, the 2018 Young Investigator Award for her research at the International Congress on Integrative Medicine and Health, and the 2017 Emerging Leader in Interprofessionalism Award at the Emswiller Interprofessional Symposium. Her research has been funded by the American Psychological Association.

Evidence to Support Mindful Healthcare Professionals

2

Kristen M. Kraemer, Amy Wang, Emily M. O'Bryan, and Christina M. Luberto

2.1 Stress-Related Problems in Healthcare Professionals

Healthcare professionals experience a myriad of stressors on the job, including challenges and demands related to patient care, administrative requirements, competing priorities, intensive work schedules, lack of control in the work setting, and high degrees of uncertainty regarding diagnosis and treatment outcomes [1–3]. As a result, healthcare professionals, such as physicians, nurses, physician assistants, pharmacists, dentists, and mental health professionals, report higher rates of stress-related problems than individuals in other professions [4–9]. One of the most concerning stress-related problems frequently endorsed by healthcare professionals is burnout, which is defined as chronic work-related stress and characterized by emotional exhaustion, depersonalization, and low personal accomplishment [10]. Burnout impacts healthcare professionals across various stages of their careers. Indeed, studies have shown that symptoms of burnout may begin as early as medical, nursing, and dental school [11–13]. Rates of burnout vary by profession but have been estimated to be as high as 80% among physicians [6], 40% among mental health professionals [4], and 26% among specialty nurses (e.g., emergency room nurses) [14] and dental staff [15].

K. M. Kraemer
Division of General Medicine, Harvard Medical School/Beth Israel Deaconess Medical Center, Boston, MA, USA
e-mail: kkraemer@bidmc.harvard.edu

A. Wang · C. M. Luberto (✉)
Department of Psychiatry, Harvard Medical School/Massachusetts General Hospital, Boston, MA, USA
e-mail: awang38@mhg.harvard.edu; cluberto@mgh.harvard.edu

E. M. O'Bryan
Anxiety Disorders Center, Institute of Living, Hartford, CT, USA
e-mail: Emily.O'Bryan@hhchealth.org

© The Author(s), under exclusive license to Springer Nature Switzerland AG 2022
S. E. Braun, P. A. Kinser (eds.), *Delivering Compassionate Care*,
https://doi.org/10.1007/978-3-030-91062-4_2

Complicating the picture, healthcare professionals are often exposed to ethical issues, institutional constraints (e.g., lack of resources, staff), traumatic events, and prolonged and intensive care of patients, resulting in feelings of moral distress and empathy fatigue [17, 18]. Moral distress, which occurs when individuals are unable to take steps they believe are right due to institutional or other constraints [18], is frequently endorsed by healthcare clinicians and is associated with higher levels of burnout and a greater intention to leave the job [17]. Empathy fatigue has been referred to as the cost of caring resulting from repeated and prolonged exposure to patient suffering [19]. Research suggests that healthcare professionals across various disciplines experience high levels of empathy fatigue [e.g., [10–22]]. Empathy fatigue is commonly referred to as "compassion fatigue" in the healthcare literature. However, it is important to consider that compassion fatigue may be a misnomer. Compassion refers to an awareness and resonance with another's suffering and a motivation to act to alleviate their suffering [23–25]. Empathy involves emotional awareness and resonance, without the added step of taking action [23–25]. As such, some researchers have suggested that the terms empathy fatigue or empathic distress may better capture the distress associated with repeated exposure to patient suffering [16, 26], as compassion may buffer against personal distress by bringing feelings of efficacy and fulfillment through the act of helping another [27, 28]. Therefore, throughout this book, we will use the more conceptually correct term of "empathy fatigue."

Burnout and empathy fatigue are associated with a number of serious job-related and personal consequences in healthcare professionals. Indeed, healthcare professional burnout has been shown to be associated with poorer quality of care (e.g., patient satisfaction) and patient safety (e.g., adverse events, medical errors) [29, 30], higher absenteeism [31], increased turnover [32], and decreased job satisfaction [32]. Furthermore, burnout has been linked to a variety of poor mental and physical health outcomes across healthcare professionals, including an increased risk of suicide in physicians [33–37]. In healthcare professional students, burnout is associated with unprofessional conduct and lower levels of empathy [38, 39]. Empathy fatigue may also be related to poorer perceived safety and quality of care [40, 41] and elevated mental health symptoms among healthcare professionals [42].

Taken together, stress-related problems (e.g., burnout, empathy fatigue) are prevalent among healthcare professionals and associated with numerous negative personal and professional consequences. Therefore, there is a critical need for interventions to prevent or mitigate the deleterious effects of stress-related problems in this vulnerable population.

2.2   Mindfulness and Compassion in Healthcare

Mindfulness-based interventions may be well-suited for addressing stress-related issues in healthcare professionals. Mindfulness, which originated in Eastern Buddhist traditions, is broadly defined as the self-regulation of attention to present moment experiences with an attitude of nonjudgment [43, 44]. The self-regulation of attention refers to deliberately directing attention to internal (i.e., thoughts, emotions, and body sensations) and external (i.e., the environment) experiences in the present moment without elaboration [45]. These experiences are then welcomed with an attitude of openness, curiosity, and acceptance [43, 46]. Inherent in mindfulness is compassion for the self (e.g., kindness toward uncomfortable experiences), which can also be applied to compassion for others through mindful social interactions. Mindfulness can refer to a state (e.g., acute attention in the present moment) [47] or a trait (e.g., dispositional tendency to be mindful in daily life) [48], with greater levels of state and trait mindfulness being associated with fewer stress-related symptoms [e.g., [49, 50]].

Mindfulness meditation practice has been shown to increase both state and trait levels of mindfulness [49, 51]. Mindfulness meditation practices, such as the body scan or awareness of breath, involve intentionally focusing on one object of awareness at a time (e.g., sensations in the body, the movement of the breath); noticing when attention has wandered from the object of focus; and gently re-directing attention back to the intended object. Each experience is observed with an attitude of curiosity and nonjudgment, allowing experiences to be as they are. Mindfulness is considered the opposite of automaticity (i.e., "automatic pilot"), which refers to the human capacity to habitually engage in behaviors without conscious awareness, or respond to experiences without deliberate intention [52]. While automaticity has its advantages, including conserving cognitive resources, automatic cognitive, emotional, and behavioral responding is associated with negative outcomes. For example, mind-wandering, an automatic cognitive process, has been linked with lower levels of happiness [53]. When experiencing high levels of stress or burnout, automatic responding is especially unlikely to be helpful, as automatic thoughts are often skewed toward negative, inaccurate perceptions of a situation, and automatic behavioral responses are based on these inaccurate thoughts rather than the situation at hand. As such, automatic responding, when stressed, tends to lead to maladaptive behavioral reactions that perpetuate and maintain emotional problems [54, 55]. Mindfulness training provides a tool to interrupt these automatic reactions by targeting the cognitive, emotional, and behavioral processes that contribute to stress and burnout, providing opportunities for more resilient outcomes (Fig. 2.1).

There are a number of interventions designed to cultivate mindfulness skills. For decades, mindfulness practices have been the interest of researchers and scholars [56]; more recently, aspects of these practices have been secularized and packaged to enhance accessibility in clinical and medical populations. Mindfulness-Based Stress Reduction (MBSR) [57] was one of the first secular mindfulness programs developed for medical settings. Since then, additional mindfulness interventions have been developed, including Mindfulness-Based Cognitive Therapy [58] and Mindful Self-Compassion [59]. Mindfulness programs are typically 8-weeks with 1–2-h sessions and daily home practice. In general, mindfulness-based interventions employ both formal (i.e., meditation, yoga) and informal practices (e.g., mindful walking, eating) to foster mindfulness skills. These interventions are designed to help build one's capacity for present moment awareness. According to theoretical frameworks underlying mindfulness interventions, efforts to avoid, change, or

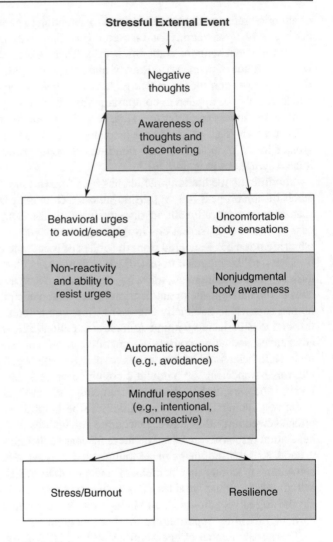

Fig. 2.1 Mindful responses versus automatic reactions to stressful external events. *Note.* White boxes indicate automatic stress reactions. Gray boxes indicate mindful responses

escape uncomfortable internal experiences (i.e., thoughts, emotions, body sensations) paradoxically maintain and exacerbate psychological distress [54, 55]. Therefore, mindfulness interventions focus on changing one's relationship with uncomfortable internal experiences (e.g., thoughts, body sensations) [60–63]. Results from several meta-analyses suggest that mindfulness-based interventions improve a variety of mental and physical health outcomes in a wide-range of populations, including symptoms of stress, anxiety, and depression [64–66], through mechanisms including trait mindfulness and more adaptive relationships to internal experiences (Fig. 2.1; e.g., decentering, non-reactivity, nonjudgment) [63, 67].

Mindfulness is closely related to compassion, which is another relevant factor in the context of healthcare. As described above, compassion is a multifaceted construct, which includes awareness that suffering is present, recognition of suffering as a common human experience, emotionally resonating with and withstanding one's own emotional reactions to the individual's suffering, and experiencing a sense of motivation to alleviate the individual's suffering [68]. Mindfulness-based interventions often include compassion meditation practices (e.g., loving-kindness meditation) and have been shown to improve several pro-social emotions, including compassion [69, 70]. Relatedly, self-compassion is linked with several positive benefits in healthcare professionals, including lower levels of caregiver fatigue and burnout and higher levels of compassion satisfaction [71–75]. There are several mindfulness-based interventions specifically developed to foster self-compassion (e.g., Mindful Self-Compassion) [59]. Overall, these and other mindfulness-based interventions have shown promise for improving levels of self-compassion [59, 76].

2.2.1   Evidence of Mindfulness Interventions for Healthcare Professionals

Mindfulness interventions have been shown effective for burnout and stress-related outcomes among healthcare professionals and students, specifically. Indeed, in a recent meta-analysis of 38 randomized controlled trials (RCTs) among a wide-range of healthcare professionals, including healthcare students/trainees, mindfulness interventions were associated with small-to-moderate improvements in symptoms of anxiety, depression, burnout, and stress [77]. Other meta-analyses have reported similar improvements in stress, burnout, and negative emotional symptoms (e.g., anxiety, depression) among various healthcare professionals [78, 79].

Extant research also suggests that mindfulness interventions may improve various indices of well-being, resilience, and pro-social emotions in healthcare professionals. For example, findings from two recent meta-analyses of mindfulness interventions demonstrated improvements in positive well-being, self-compassion, and trait levels of mindfulness among mixed samples of healthcare professionals and students [77, 79]. Wasson and colleagues [80] conducted a meta-analysis of 27 studies examining the effects of mindfulness interventions on self-compassion in healthcare professionals and students. Overall, there were moderate effects at post-intervention and follow-up, suggesting that mindfulness interventions are effective for improving self-compassion in this population. Although more research is needed, there is preliminary evidence that mindfulness interventions may improve empathy in physicians [81], nurses [82], and healthcare students [83].

Compassion-focused interventions, which commonly include loving-kindness practices, have also shown promise for healthcare professionals. Non-randomized studies suggest that compassion-focused interventions may improve indices of self-compassion, mindfulness skills, stress, burnout, and resilience among various healthcare professionals [84], including palliative care teams [85], nurses [86], and medical students [87]. Research indicates that integrating loving-kindness practices with other mind-body skills may also improve stress-related outcomes, indices of resilience, and confidence providing compassionate care in various healthcare professionals and trainees [88–90]. In one of the few randomized controlled trials to date, medical students who completed compassion training reported increases in compassion and decreases in loneliness and depression [91].

There is also preliminary evidence for self-compassion focused mindfulness interventions for healthcare workers. For example, in a small pilot study, Mindful Self-Compassion resulted in improvements in secondary trauma, burnout, resilience, and compassion satisfaction among nurses [92]. In a second study among various healthcare professionals, Neff and colleagues [93] found that Mindful Self-Compassion training led to improvements in self-compassion, well-being, secondary traumatic stress, and burnout.

Importantly, mindfulness interventions for healthcare professionals have also shown promise for improving patient care-related outcomes. Braun and colleagues [94] synthesized the research on mindfulness for several patient care outcomes. Overall, results from 26 studies provided strong evidence for the effects of mindfulness on healthcare professional-reported patient care (e.g., confidence in providing care), moderate evidence for patient safety, patient treatment outcomes, and patient-centered care, and weak evidence for patient satisfaction. To guide future research in this area, Braun and colleagues [94] developed a theoretical framework (see Fig. 2.2), which proposes that mindfulness interventions may improve patient care related outcomes through healthcare provider improvements in emotional competency, cognitive function, and burnout.

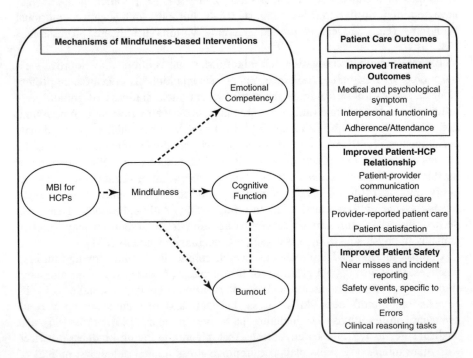

Fig. 2.2 Proposed mechanisms of mindfulness-based interventions for patient care (reprinted with permission from Braun, Kinser, & Rybarczyk, 2019)

2.2.2 Mindfulness for Interdisciplinary Healthcare Professionals

One particular program that has received empirical attention is Mindfulness for Interdisciplinary Healthcare Professionals (MIHP). MIHP is an 8-week mindfulness program, based on the format of MBSR, that was designed specifically for healthcare professionals. Each 2-h group session focuses on applying mindfulness in the context of healthcare work, with half of the session focused on discussion and didactics related to the session theme (e.g., mindfulness for burnout and managing suffering, mindful leadership), and the other half dedicated to experiential mindfulness practices (e.g., yoga, seated meditation).

In an early pilot study, MIHP was found to be feasible and acceptable for healthcare professionals and trainees across disciplines (e.g., nursing, dentistry, psychiatry) [95]. Preliminary data suggested that MIHP was associated with improvements in perceived stress, anxiety symptoms, and the emotional exhaustion component of burnout. Furthermore, improvements in burnout and dispositional mindfulness were maintained over a long-term follow-up period (6–18 months) [96]. Qualitative data suggests that participants in MIHP emphasized the importance of integrating mindfulness practices into their daily lives, valued the informal mindfulness practices more than the formal practices (e.g., seated meditations) due to time constraints, and noted that mindfulness was a helpful tool to foster connections with the self, others, and patients [96]. In a recent study among healthcare professional students, compared to a waitlist group, participants in MIHP demonstrated improvements in burnout, perceived stress, trait mindfulness, and daily activity impairment due to physical/mental health issues, but not cognitive performance or work productivity [97].

2.3 Conclusions

Taken together, mindfulness interventions are well-suited for addressing the high rates of stress-related problems among healthcare professionals. Mindfulness interventions have been shown to be beneficial for improving stress, burnout, self-compassion, and overall well-being across various healthcare professions. MIHP is one evidence-based mindfulness program designed specifically for healthcare professionals that has demonstrated promise for reducing stress-related symptoms. As discussed throughout this book, this MIHP curriculum provides an opportunity for healthcare professionals to explore mindfulness practices for their personal use with the potential for downstream effects on patient care.

References

1. Patel RS, Bachu R, Adikey A, Malik M, Shah M. Factors related to physician burnout and its consequences: a review. Behav Sci. 2018;8:98.
2. Simpkin AL, Schwartzstein RM. Tolerating uncertainty—the next medical revolution? N Engl J Med. 2016;375:1713–5.

3. Van Bogaert P, Peremans L, Van Heusden D, Verspuy M, Kureckova V, Van de Cruys Z, et al. Predictors of burnout, work engagement and nurse reported job outcomes and quality of care: a mixed method study. BMC Nurs. 2017;16:1–4.
4. O'Connor K, Neff DM, Pitman S. Burnout in mental health professionals: a systematic review and meta-analysis of prevalence and determinants. Eur Psychiatry. 2018;53:74–99.
5. McQuade BM, Reed BN, DiDomenico RJ, Baker WL, Shipper AG, Jarrett JB. Feeling the burn? A systematic review of burnout in pharmacists. J Am Coll Clin Pharm. 2020;3:663–75.
6. Rotenstein LS, Torre M, Ramos MA, Rosales RC, Guille C, Sen S, et al. Prevalence of burnout among physicians: a systematic review. JAMA. 2018;320:1131–50.
7. Tetzlaff ED, Hylton HM, DeMora L, Ruth K, Wong YN. National study of burnout and career satisfaction among physician assistants in oncology: implications for team-based care. J Oncol Pract. 2018;14:e11–22.
8. Woo T, Ho R, Tang A, Tam W. Global prevalence of burnout symptoms among nurses: a systematic review and meta-analysis. J Psychiatr Res. 2020;123:9–20.
9. Singh P, Aulak DS, Mangat SS, Aulak MS. Systematic review: factors contributing to burnout in dentistry. Occup Med. 2016;66:27–31.
10. Maslach C, Leiter MP. Understanding the burnout experience: recent research and its implications for psychiatry. World Psychiatry. 2016;15:103–11.
11. Frajerman A, Morvan Y, Krebs MO, Gorwood P, Chaumette B. Burnout in medical students before residency: a systematic review and meta-analysis. Eur Psychiatry. 2019;55:36–42.
12. Pöhlmann K, Jonas I, Ruf S, Harzer W. Stress, burnout and health in the clinical period of dental education. Eur J Dent Educ. 2005;9:78–84.
13. Rella S, Winwood PC, Lushington K. When does nursing burnout begin? An investigation of the fatigue experience of Australian nursing students. J Nurs Manag. 2009;17:886–97.
14. Adriaenssens J, De Gucht V, Maes S. Determinants and prevalence of burnout in emergency nurses: a systematic review of 25 years of research. Int J Nurs Stud. 2015;52:649–61.
15. Gorter RC, Freeman R. Burnout and engagement in relation with job demands and resources among dental staff in Northern Ireland. Community Dent Oral Epidemiol. 2011;39:87–95.
16. Sinclair S, Raffin-Bouchal S, Venturato L, Mijovic-Kondejewski J, Smith-MacDonald L. Compassion fatigue: a meta-narrative review of the healthcare literature. Int J Nurs Stud. 2017;69:9–24.
17. Whitehead PB, Herbertson RK, Hamric AB, Epstein EG, Fisher JM. Moral distress among healthcare professionals: report of an institution-wide survey. J Nurs Scholarsh. 2015;47:117–25.
18. Jameton A. Dilemmas of moral distress: moral responsibility and nursing practice. AWHONNs Clin Issues Perinat Womens Health Nurs. 1993;4:542–51.
19. Figley CR. Compassion fatigue: psychotherapists' chronic lack of self care. J Clin Psychol. 2002;58:1433–41.
20. Gribben JL, Kase SM, Waldman ED, Weintraub AS. A cross-sectional analysis of compassion fatigue, burnout, and compassion satisfaction in pediatric critical care physicians in the United States. Pediatr Crit Care Med. 2019;20:213–22.
21. Nolte AG, Downing C, Temane A, Hastings-Tolsma M. Compassion fatigue in nurses: a meta-synthesis. J Clin Nurs. 2017;26:4364–78.
22. Pelon SB. Compassion fatigue and compassion satisfaction in hospice social work. J Soc Work End Life Palliat Care. 2017;13:134–50.
23. Keltner D, Goetz JL. In: Baumeister RF, Vohs KD, editors. Encyclopedia of social psychology. Thousand Oaks: Sage; 2007. p. 159–61.
24. Klimecki OM, Leiberg S, Ricard M, Singer T. Differential pattern of functional brain plasticity after compassion and empathy training. Soc Cogn Affect Neurosci. 2014;9:873–9.
25. Singer T, Klimecki OM. Empathy and compassion. Curr Biol. 2014;24:R875–8.
26. Hofmeyer A, Kennedy K, Taylor R. Contesting the term 'compassion fatigue': integrating findings from social neuroscience and self-care research. Collegian. 2020;27:232–7.
27. Goetz JL, Keltner D, Simon-Thomas E. Compassion: an evolutionary analysis and empirical review. Psychol Bull. 2010;136:351–74.

28. Klimecki O, Singer T. Empathic distress fatigue rather than compassion fatigue? Integrating findings from empathy research in psychology and social neuroscience. In: Oakley B, Knafo A, Madhavan G, Sloan Wilson G, editors. Pathological altruism. New York: Oxford University Press; 2012. p. 368–83.
29. Panagioti M, Geraghty K, Johnson J, Zhou A, Panagopoulou E, Chew-Graham C, et al. Association between physician burnout and patient safety, professionalism, and patient satisfaction: a systematic review and meta-analysis. JAMA Intern Med. 2018;178:1317–31.
30. Salyers MP, Bonfils KA, Luther L, Firmin RL, White DA, Adams EL, et al. The relationship between professional burnout and quality and safety in healthcare: a meta-analysis. J Gen Intern Med. 2017;32:475–82.
31. Dyrbye LN, Shanafelt TD, Johnson PO, Johnson LA, Satele D, West CP. A cross-sectional study exploring the relationship between burnout, absenteeism, and job performance among American nurses. BMC Nurs. 2019;18:1–8.
32. Scanlan JN, Still M. Relationships between burnout, turnover intention, job satisfaction, job demands and job resources for mental health personnel in an Australian mental health service. BMC Health Serv Res. 2019;19:1–1.
33. Embriaco N, Papazian L, Kentish-Barnes N, Pochard F, Azoulay E. Burnout syndrome among critical care healthcare workers. Curr Opin Crit Care. 2007;13:482–8.
34. Khamisa N, Peltzer K, Oldenburg B. Burnout in relation to specific contributing factors and health outcomes among nurses: a systematic review. Int J Environ Res Public Health. 2013;10:2214–40.
35. Peterson U, Demerouti E, Bergström G, Samuelsson M, Åsberg M, Nygren Å. Burnout and physical and mental health among Swedish healthcare workers. J Adv Nurs. 2008;62:84–95.
36. Shanafelt TD, Balch CM, Dyrbye L, Bechamps G, Russell T, Satele D, et al. Special report: suicidal ideation among American surgeons. Arch Surg. 2011;146:54–62.
37. Van der Heijden F, Dillingh G, Bakker A, Prins J. Suicidal thoughts among medical residents with burnout. Arch Suicide Res. 2008;12:344–6.
38. Dyrbye LN, Massie FS, Eacker A, Harper W, Power D, Durning SJ, et al. Relationship between burnout and professional conduct and attitudes among US medical students. JAMA. 2010;304:1173–80.
39. Paro HB, Silveira PS, Perotta B, Gannam S, Enns SC, Giaxa RR, et al. Empathy among medical students: is there a relation with quality of life and burnout? PLoS One. 2014;9:e94133.
40. Maiden J, Georges JM, Connelly CD. Moral distress, compassion fatigue, and perceptions about medication errors in certified critical care nurses. Dimens Crit Care Nurs. 2011;30:339–45.
41. Slatten LA, Carson KD, Carson PP. Compassion fatigue and burnout: what managers should know. Health Care Manag. 2011;30(4):325–33.
42. Hegney DG, Craigie M, Hemsworth D, Osseiran-Moisson R, Aoun S, Francis K, et al. Compassion satisfaction, compassion fatigue, anxiety, depression and stress in registered nurses in Australia: study 1 results. J Nurs Manag. 2014;22:506–18.
43. Bishop SR, Lau M, Shapiro S, Carlson L, Anderson ND, Carmody J, et al. Mindfulness: a proposed operational definition. Clin Psychol (New York). 2004;11:230–41.
44. Kabat-Zinn J. Wherever you go, there you are: mindfulness meditation in everyday life. New York: Hachette Books; 2009.
45. Teasdale JD, Segal Z, Williams JM. How does cognitive therapy prevent depressive relapse and why should attentional control (mindfulness) training help? Behav Res Ther. 1995;33:25–39.
46. Kabat-Zinn J. Mindfulness-based interventions in context: past, present, and future. Clin Psychol (New York). 2003;10:144–56.
47. Lau MA, Bishop SR, Segal ZV, Buis T, Anderson ND, Carlson L, et al. The Toronto mindfulness scale: development and validation. J Clin Psychol. 2006;62:1445–67.
48. Baer RA, Smith GT, Hopkins J, Krietemeyer J, Toney L. Using self-report assessment methods to explore facets of mindfulness. Assessment. 2006;13:27–45.
49. Kiken LG, Garland EL, Bluth K, Palsson OS, Gaylord SA. From a state to a trait: trajectories of state mindfulness in meditation during intervention predict changes in trait mindfulness. Pers Individ Dif. 2015;81:41–6.

50. Tomlinson ER, Yousaf O, Vittersø AD, Jones L. Dispositional mindfulness and psychological health: a systematic review. Mindfulness. 2018;9:23–43.
51. Quaglia JT, Braun SE, Freeman SP, McDaniel MA, Brown KW. Meta-analytic evidence for effects of mindfulness training on dimensions of self-reported dispositional mindfulness. Psychol Assess. 2016;28:803–18.
52. Kang Y, Gruber J, Gray JR. Mindfulness and de-automatization. Emot Rev. 2013;5:192–201.
53. Killingsworth MA, Gilbert DT. A wandering mind is an unhappy mind. Science. 2010;330:932.
54. Brown KW, Ryan RM, Creswell JD. Mindfulness: theoretical foundations and evidence for its salutary effects. Psychol Inq. 2007;18:211–37.
55. Hayes SC. Acceptance and commitment therapy, relational frame theory, and the third wave of behavioral and cognitive therapies. Behav Ther. 2004;35:639–65.
56. Siegel RD, Germer CK, Olendzki A. Mindfulness: what is it? Where did it come from? In: Didonna F, editor. Clinical handbook of mindfulness. New York: Springer; 2009. p. 17–35.
57. Kabat-Zinn J. An outpatient program in behavioral medicine for chronic pain patients based on the practice of mindfulness meditation: theoretical considerations and preliminary results. Gen Hosp Psychiatry. 1982;4:33–47.
58. Segal ZV, Williams M, Teasdale J. Mindfulness-based cognitive therapy for depression. 2nd ed. New York: Guilford Publications; 2018.
59. Neff KD, Germer CK. A pilot study and randomized controlled trial of the mindful self-compassion program. J Clin Psychol. 2013;69:28–44.
60. Hoge EA, Bui E, Goetter E, Robinaugh DJ, Ojserkis RA, Fresco DM, et al. Change in decentering mediates improvement in anxiety in mindfulness-based stress reduction for generalized anxiety disorder. Cogn Ther Res. 2015;39:228–35.
61. Hölzel BK, Lazar SW, Gard T, Schuman-Olivier Z, Vago DR, Ott U. How does mindfulness meditation work? Proposing mechanisms of action from a conceptual and neural perspective. Perspect Psychol Sci. 2011;6:537–59.
62. Lindsay EK, Creswell JD. Mechanisms of mindfulness training: monitor and acceptance theory (MAT). Clin Psychol Rev. 2017;51:48–59.
63. Sauer S, Baer RA. Mindfulness and decentering as mechanisms of change in mindfulness-and acceptance-based interventions. In: Baer RA, editor. Assessing mindfulness and acceptance processes in clients. Oakland: Context Press; 2010. p. 25–50.
64. Grossman P, Niemann L, Schmidt S, Walach H. Mindfulness-based stress reduction and health benefits: a meta-analysis. J Psychosom Res. 2004;57:35–43.
65. Hofmann SG, Sawyer AT, Witt AA, Oh D. The effect of mindfulness-based therapy on anxiety and depression: a meta-analytic review. J Consult Clin Psychol. 2010;78:169–83.
66. Vøllestad J, Nielsen MB, Nielsen GH. Mindfulness-and acceptance-based interventions for anxiety disorders: a systematic review and meta-analysis. Br J Clin Psychol. 2012;51:239–60.
67. Gu J, Strauss C, Bond R, Cavanagh K. How do mindfulness-based cognitive therapy and mindfulness-based stress reduction improve mental health and wellbeing? A systematic review and meta-analysis of mediation studies. Clin Psychol Rev. 2015 Apr;1(37):1–2.
68. Strauss C, Taylor BL, Gu J, Kuyken W, Baer R, Jones F, Cavanagh K. What is compassion and how can we measure it? A review of definitions and measures. Clin Psychol Rev. 2016;47:15–27.
69. Chiesa A, Serretti A. Mindfulness-based stress reduction for stress management in healthy people: a review and meta-analysis. J Altern Complement Med. 2009;15:593–600.
70. Luberto CM, Shinday N, Song R, Philpotts LL, Park ER, Fricchione GL, et al. A systematic review and meta-analysis of the effects of meditation on empathy, compassion, and prosocial behaviors. Mindfulness. 2018;9:708–24.
71. Atkinson DM, Rodman JL, Thuras PD, Shiroma PR, Lim KO. Examining burnout, depression, and self-compassion in veterans affairs mental health staff. J Altern Complement Med. 2017;23:551–7.
72. Beaumont E, Durkin M, Martin CJ, Carson J. Compassion for others, self-compassion, quality of life and mental well-being measures and their association with compassion fatigue and burnout in student midwives: a quantitative survey. Midwifery. 2016;34:239–44.

73. Duarte J, Pinto-Gouveia J, Cruz B. Relationships between nurses' empathy, self-compassion and dimensions of professional quality of life: a cross-sectional study. Int J Nurs Stud. 2016;60:1–1.
74. Durkin M, Beaumont E, Martin CJ, Carson J. A pilot study exploring the relationship between self-compassion, self-judgement, self-kindness, compassion, professional quality of life and wellbeing among UK community nurses. Nurse Educ Today. 2016;46:109–14.
75. Olson K, Kemper KJ, Mahan JD. What factors promote resilience and protect against burnout in first-year pediatric and medicine-pediatric residents? Evid Based Complement Alternat Med. 2015;20(3):192–8.
76. Ferrari M, Hunt C, Harrysunker A, Abbott MJ, Beath AP, Einstein DA. Self-compassion interventions and psychosocial outcomes: a meta-analysis of RCTs. Mindfulness. 2019;10:1455–73.
77. Spinelli C, Wisener M, Khoury B. Mindfulness training for healthcare professionals and trainees: a meta-analysis of randomized controlled trials. J Psychosom Res. 2019;120:29–38.
78. Burton A, Burgess C, Dean S, Koutsopoulou GZ, Hugh-Jones S. How effective are mindfulness-based interventions for reducing stress among healthcare professionals? A systematic review and meta-analysis. Stress Health. 2017;33:3–13.
79. Lomas T, Medina JC, Ivtzan I, Rupprecht S, Eiroa-Orosa FJ. A systematic review and meta-analysis of the impact of mindfulness-based interventions on the well-being of healthcare professionals. Mindfulness. 2019;10:1193–216.
80. Wasson RS, Barratt C, O'Brien WH. Effects of mindfulness-based interventions on self-compassion in health care professionals: a meta-analysis. Mindfulness. 2020;11:1914–34.
81. Krasner MS, Epstein RM, Beckman H, Suchman AL, Chapman B, Mooney CJ, et al. Association of an educational program in mindful communication with burnout, empathy, and attitudes among primary care physicians. JAMA. 2009;302:1284–93.
82. Bazarko D, Cate RA, Azocar F, Kreitzer MJ. The impact of an innovative mindfulness-based stress reduction program on the health and well-being of nurses employed in a corporate setting. J Workplace Behav Health. 2013;28:107–33.
83. Barbosa P, Raymond G, Zlotnick C, Wilk J, Toomey R III, Mitchell J III. Mindfulness-based stress reduction training is associated with greater empathy and reduced anxiety for graduate healthcare students. Educ Health. 2013;26:9–14.
84. Scarlet J, Altmeyer N, Knier S, Harpin RE. The effects of compassion cultivation training (CCT) on health-care workers. Clin Psychol. 2017;21:116–24.
85. Orellana-Rios CL, Radbruch L, Kern M, Regel YU, Anton A, Sinclair S, Schmidt S. Mindfulness and compassion-oriented practices at work reduce distress and enhance self-care of palliative care teams: a mixed-method evaluation of an "on the job" program. BMC Palliat. 2018;17:1–5.
86. dos Santos TM, Kozasa EH, Carmagnani IS, Tanaka LH, Lacerda SS, Nogueira-Martins LA. Positive effects of a stress reduction program based on mindfulness meditation in Brazilian nursing professionals: qualitative and quantitative evaluation. Explore. 2016;12:90–9.
87. Weingartner LA, Sawning S, Shaw MA, Klein JB. Compassion cultivation training promotes medical student wellness and enhanced clinical care. BMC Med Educ. 2019;19:139.
88. Kemper KJ, Lynn J, Mahan JD. What is the impact of online training in mind–body skills? J Evid Based Complement Alternat Med. 2015;20:275–82.
89. Kemper KJ, Khirallah M. Acute effects of online mind–body skills training on resilience, mindfulness, and empathy. J Evid Based Complement Alternat Med. 2015;20:247–53.
90. Rao N, Kemper KJ. Online training in specific meditation practices improves gratitude, well-being, self-compassion, and confidence in providing compassionate care among health professionals. J Evid Based Complement Alternat Med. 2017;22:237–41.
91. Mascaro JS, Kelley S, Darcher A, Negi LT, Worthman C, Miller A, Raison C. Meditation buffers medical student compassion from the deleterious effects of depression. J Posit Psychol. 2018;13:133–42.
92. Delaney MC. Caring for the caregivers: evaluation of the effect of an eight-week pilot mindful self-compassion (MSC) training program on nurses' compassion fatigue and resilience. PLoS One. 2018;13(11):e0207261.

93. Neff KD, Knox MC, Long P, Gregory K. Caring for others without losing yourself: an adaptation of the mindful self-compassion program for healthcare communities. J Clin Psychol. 2020;76:1543–62.
94. Braun SE, Kinser PA, Rybarczyk B. Can mindfulness in health care professionals improve patient care? An integrative review and proposed model. Transl Behav Med. 2019;9:187–201.
95. Kinser P, Braun S, Deeb G, Carrico C, Dow A. "Awareness is the first step": an interprofessional course on mindfulness & mindful-movement for healthcare professionals and students. Complement Ther Clin Pract. 2016;25:18–25.
96. Braun SE, Kinser P, Carrico CK, Dow A. Being mindful: a long-term investigation of an interdisciplinary course in mindfulness. Glob Adv Health Med. 2019;8:2164956118820064.
97. Braun SE, Dow A, Loughan A, Mladen S, Crawford M, Rybarczyk B, Kinser, P. Mindfulness training for healthcare professional students: a waitlist controlled pilot study on psychological and work-relevant outcomes. Complement Ther Med. 2020;51:102405.

Compassionate Healthcare

3

Sarah Ellen Braun and Jordan Quaglia

3.1 Compassion Training for the Healthcare Professional

Compassion can be defined as the acknowledgment and desire to relieve another's suffering. A related term and practice, loving kindness, is the act of wishing happiness and freedom toward another. There has been increased interest in the secularization of practices that train compassion, which originate in Buddhist philosophy. While we will not fully delve into the Buddhist origins of compassion, we do think a brief explanation of compassion from the Buddhist perspective is important for framing how it can be helpful for healthcare professionals, and understanding how the teachings of compassion have changed in their secular presentation. From certain Buddhist traditions, the desire to relieve suffering for all beings is a fundamental goal of the practitioner. Training and cultivating compassion are integral to this practice. In this framework, the Buddhist practitioner devotes their life and practice in service of others, specifically to actively work toward freedom from suffering for all beings. A wonderful chapter on how specific Buddhist perspectives have influenced modern secular compassion interventions can be found in Lavelle 2017 [1].

In this manual, as well as in other compassion trainings for the healthcare professional, the spiritual philosophy has been underemphasized, if not removed, to make the teachings more generalizable. From the secular perspective presented here, compassion is an emotion and practice that can be cultivated to optimize our capacity to sit with suffering, whether our own and that of others. In this way it improves our ability to manage stressful situations as well as to provide patient-centered care. This distinction is important because, from the secular perspective, compassion is

S. E. Braun (✉)
Department of Neurology, School of Medicine, Virginia Commonwealth University, Richmond, VA, USA
e-mail: sarah.braun@vcuhealth.org

J. Quaglia
Naropa University, Boulder, CO, USA

not only about supporting others. Rather, it can support us personally in improving ourselves, our abilities, and our work. As you read through this chapter and manual, we encourage you to keep in the mind that these practices help us find an optimal balance between caring for ourselves and others. Ultimately, we prefer to think of mindfulness and compassion as parts of the inner work needed to be of service to others sustainably, over the long term.

3.2   The Relationality of Compassion

In our view, compassion is an inherently relational quality, consistent with the perspective outlined by Condon and Makransky 2020 [2]. This means that through the practice of compassion we move through several teachings which help us navigate our interdependence with others. This may be particularly relevant for healthcare professionals because we aim to develop unconditional compassion—for all beings, regardless of who they are or what they have done. In so doing, we are able to access a deeper source of compassion for others—a necessary skill for our jobs which regularly expose us to the extremes of human suffering and the fullness of humanity. Our manual trains both mindfulness and compassion, as both are deemed essential for the healthcare professional. We begin with mindfulness—training the mind to be present to reality as it arises. From there, we begin to cultivate loving-kindness and compassion, first toward ourselves, then toward a loved one, then someone neutral, and then toward someone for whom these feelings are difficult to cultivate. Eventually, we develop loving-kindness and compassion for all beings. Finally, we practice what can be called "active compassion" through a practice called tonglen or "sending and receiving," in which we envision taking on the suffering of others and sending it out, transformed, as freedom and relief. In the 8-week course, we introduce and encourage each of these practices, in this order, but we also invite practitioners to develop their own home practice with the specific practices that resonate with them. Said simply, we present a variety of tools and perspectives— you decide what works for you.

It is important to distinguish compassion from a self-help tool, which over emphasizes an individualistic idea of compassion. Instead, compassion is fundamentally about connection. The ability to feel compassion toward another comes from a place of security and safety that is supported by our connection to others, to our own suffering, and to our acknowledgment that suffering is an aspect of human experience shared by everyone. Mindfulness and compassion are connected to one another in this way. Through mindfulness practices, like focused attention meditation, we train the ability to be aware of reality as it arises. This invariably introduces us to our own suffering in deeper and clearer ways. If we exclusively practice mindfulness, honing our awareness to greater degrees, then we may find ourselves with a deeper awareness of suffering, but without a container in which to hold it. Therein lies the role of compassion. When we train compassion, we begin with a practice of feeling loved, safe, and secure. There are different practices to elicit these feelings, including loving-kindness, which is discussed below. By beginning here, we connect to the innate desire in ourselves to be happy and content and create an internal pathway to feel connected, supported, and safe. From this place, we begin to train compassion toward others, toward all sentient beings, including ourselves. This process begins with an awareness of our suffering, which acts as a portal, connecting us to others through the shared experience of suffering.

The process by which we train compassion gently lessens the learned neurosis and biases that maintain a sense of disconnection from others. While the concepts of mindfulness and compassion are presented in various ways, our approach seeks to restructure these concepts as part of a "relational foundation" as described by Condon and Makransky [2]. Accordingly, mindfulness and compassion training both come from a place of connection with others. We are not on our own. We are not meditating in a vacuum in order to feel better about ourselves. To the contrary, these practices are fundamentally about cultivating a healthy balance of care for self and others. When we approach them purely as a form of self-help—or alternatively, self-sacrifice—we run the risk of more firmly establishing a sense of self-importance, cognitive rigidity, and, even as we will discuss, burnout.

3.3 Compassion Includes Self-Compassion

Because of the inherent relationality of compassion, we typically recommend thinking about self-compassion and other-oriented compassion together, as two inherently connected sides of compassion as a whole [3]. There are some scholars and practitioners who tend to emphasize one orientation of compassion or another (e.g., Neff, 2003) [4], but this is mostly for pragmatic purposes. Most scholars agree that compassion directed toward the self is not the full experience of compassion, and neither is compassion directed solely toward others. To maximize the benefits of compassion, it is important to experience and train in both self-compassion and other compassion. This said, self-compassion may be helpful to experience the felt sense of acknowledging and wishing to relieve suffering, and so can be a doorway to connecting with the suffering of others. Similarly, the practice of other compassion can help us recognize ourselves in others—and therefore that we, too, deserve our own care and affection. With that said, the specific practices of compassion that are taught in this manual begin with offering loving-kindness and compassion to the self, followed by increasingly more distal and larger groups of "others," eventually offering compassion to all beings. This sequence of compassion is one way to train and grow the concept of compassion and may be particularly useful for training compassion in individualistic cultures, by beginning with the self. Nevertheless, there are other ways to train compassion and the focus of a compassion meditation can be adapted to any person, group, or being. In this way, compassion training blends the self and other and develops connection with all beings via the experience of suffering.

3.4 Compassion Is Innate

Perhaps you consider compassion to be something that people experience naturally. Indeed, for most healthcare professionals, compassion may be what motivated them to pursue a career in caring for others. Consistent with this perspective, most scientists agree that compassion *is* innate (cf. Goetz et al., 2010) [5]. Why, then, do we rely on practices to cultivate compassion? For most of us, it is innate to feel compassion for our children, our families, and our loved ones. But compassion for others—those for whom we are neutral toward, those who are in an "outgroup," and those who may have hurt us or threatened to hurt us—is more challenging. Therefore, to cultivate the kind of compassion we talk about here—and that applies to the context of working with patients who are not part of our natural circle of care—it is important to grow and extend our compassion through compassion training. At more advanced levels of compassion training, our compassion can even grow to be unconditional, including those for whom we may not "like" in the conventional sense. Even if someone has caused harm to us or others, we can come to recognize their own suffering as the source of their harmful actions, and thereby consider what may help them experience freedom from that suffering and the harm it creates. While not always easy, we can learn to grow our compassion in ways that include all beings.

3.5 Compassionate Healthcare

The everyday work of healthcare professionals (HCPs) is distinguished in part by the heightened presence of others' suffering. Compared with many other professions, HCPs face greater frequency, duration, and intensity of others' suffering while at work. Given this, it is not surprising that HCPs are at risk for experiences such as empathic distress, vicarious trauma, and burnout. Indeed, controlling for other factors, HCPs are at twice the risk for burnout compared to the general population [6]. Yet a mindful approach to healthcare acknowledges that awareness has power. Recognizing the inevitability of encountering others' pain, distress, and suffering gives us the chance to prepare our minds and hearts, just as we may prepare for other aspects of the job. As we explore in this chapter, the cultivation of both mindfulness and compassion can act as a kind of inner preparation for recurrent exposure to suffering in healthcare settings. Indeed, both factors—and their combination in mindful compassion—are uniquely suited for the demands that others' suffering place on HCPs. This is because, unlikely many other strategies, the orientation of mindful compassion toward suffering is rooted in approach rather than avoidance. Put another way, mindful compassion involves growing our awareness of suffering—whether in ourselves or others—rather than trying to ignore, suppress, or otherwise minimize its presence.

Perhaps the best way to appreciate the benefits of mindful compassion is through exploring the distinction between compassion and empathy. People often conflate empathy and compassion, using them interchangeably. This is true, it seems, even for many professionals who work in this area. For example, the phrase *compassion fatigue* has been popularized in the scientific literature [7], leading to burgeoning literature on the phenomenon of exhaustion and related feelings that can arise in care providers due to chronic engagement with empathy for the suffering [8]. Yet, as others have pointed out in the scientific literature [9], the phenomenon is actually more akin to *empathy fatigue*, since the reported symptoms of compassion fatigue are more consistent with the downsides of empathy and empathy avoidance [9].

One reason for this confusion may be that empathy serves as a precursor for compassion. Specifically, when we empathize with others suffering, we experience the first step of compassion. This tends to be a relatively subconscious and automatic experience—human beings are hardwired to not only discern, but also simulate, the internal states of others within their own body and mind [10]. What's more, people often engage in some kind of effortful avoidance of empathy due to perceived costs such as pain and task interference [11]. This effortful avoidance of something that is quite automatic and natural means that the conscious mind must intervene to override the empathic response, leading to an exhausting, internal tug-of-war with our own innate tendencies. Consequently, empathy and its avoidance can tax our limited bioenergetic resources, leading to empathy fatigue.

What, then, distinguishes compassion from empathy? Said simply, empathy is more about feeling *with* what others are feeling, whereas compassion is more about feeling *for* what others are feeling [12]. Compassion takes empathy for suffering as its starting point, but ultimately transforms empathy into a more conscious, regulated experience. Generally, researchers consider three components to be primary to compassion, namely (1) greater awareness of suffering, (2) feeling for the one who is suffering, and (3) an intentional readiness to alleviate suffering if possible [13, 14]. Compassion has thus been understood as having essential cognitive, affective, and motivational components. These essential aspects are summarized succinctly by the Dalai Lama's [15] definition of other-oriented compassion as, "An openness to the suffering of others with a commitment to relieve it." Compassion practices and training work to directly support and train these three components, thereby increasing the frequency, duration, and strength of their deployment in daily life.

In the presence of suffering, this compassionate orientation therefore works with, rather than against, our natural empathy. This is because the three components of compassion ensure that our awareness of suffering does not remain subconscious, and that our habitual avoidance mechanisms do not exhaust our mental resources. The result of this more conscious stance toward suffering is that compassion becomes an important protective factor against empathy fatigue and its close cousin, burnout. This protective aspect of compassion is made even stronger when we train in mindfulness as well, since mindfulness supports breaking habits generally, including our habits for avoiding, suppressing, or minimizing suffering.

Although scientific research on mindfulness and compassion is still fairly new, these internal factors have long been recognized as a kind of buffer against exhaustion and burnout when working to alleviate suffering in the world. From this perspective, their cultivation may be even more important for HCPs than for those who work in other settings, where suffering is not as pronounced. As part of a broader strategy that includes attention to external factors, the protective internal factors of mindfulness and compassion should give us hope for the well-being of HCPs. The growing body of research on them underscore how greater HCP suffering need not be an inevitable aspect of their frequent encounters with the suffering of others. Moreover, the trainable nature of mindful compassion means HCPs can be proactive in training to decrease the likelihood of empathy fatigue and burnout.

3.6   Training Compassion

There are three types of practices introduced throughout this manual that train compassion. First, we start with loving-kindness meditation, which serves to develop feelings of connection and wishing happiness and safety for others. Then, we practice compassion meditation, to acknowledge suffering and develop a strong desire to end suffering and its causes for all beings. Finally, we practice tonglen, which is a visualization of transforming suffering. In this manual, we teach all of these practices by beginning with a focus on the self, then moving the focus outward until it encompasses all sentient beings. Loving-kindness and compassion meditation are taught in this manual in a holistic way, using common phrases to offer loving-kindness and compassion to the self, a close loved-one, a neutral person, someone difficult, and then all beings.

Consistent with compassion generally, tonglen practice asks us to approach—rather than avoid—the difficult, the dark, and the suffering of our world. By leaning into this suffering, we are able to not only face suffering more fully, but we also transform the suffering into healing, and share this potential of compassion with the world. When teaching tonglen, it is important to acknowledge that this practice is a form of active compassion that readies us to take action, off the cushion, to relieve the suffering of others. Tonglen therefore prepares us to approach the suffering in our lives and that of others with greater regulation, curiosity, and deeper motivation to be of service to those suffering. It is also important to note that the practice of tonglen may be more difficult than other compassion practices, as it asks us to visualize taking on the suffering of others and to transform that into freedom and relief. Fortunately, tonglen reminds us that we do not do this alone. In practicing tonglen, we connect with the strength and wisdom of all the people who have delved into these practices before us, as well as others who engage these practices now. Tonglen may therefore be thought of as a more advanced compassion practice Accordingly, when teaching tonglen, it is important to remind your students that it can be a powerful practice, and to encourage discussion and questions as needed. Most essential, in our view, is for an instructor to have an established practice of tonglen prior to teaching it to others [16].

References

1. Dodson-Lavelle B. Compassion in context: tracing the Buddhist roots of secular, compassion-based contemplative programs. In: The Oxford handbook compassion science. Oxford: Oxford University Press; 2017.

2. Condon P, Makransky J. Recovering the relational starting point of compassion training: a foundation for sustainable and inclusive care. Perspect Psychol Sci. 2020;15(6):1346–62.
3. Quaglia JT, Soisson A, Simmer-Brown J. Compassion for self versus other: a critical review of compassion training research. J Posit Psychol. 2021;16(5):675–90. https://doi.org/10.108 0/17439760.2020.1805502.
4. Neff KD. The development and validation of a scale to measure self-compassion. Self Identity. 2003;2(3):223–50.
5. Goetz JL, Keltner D, Simon-Thomas E. Compassion: an evolutionary analysis and empirical review. Psychol Bull. 2010;136(3):351.
6. Shanafelt TD, Boone S, Tan L, Dyrbye LN, Sotile W, Satele D, et al. Burnout and satisfaction with work-life balance among US physicians relative to the general US population. Arch Intern Med. 2012;172(18):1377. http://www.ncbi.nlm.nih.gov/pubmed/22911330%5Cn, http://archinte.jamanetwork.com/data/Journals/INTEMED/25300/ioi120042_1377_1385.pdf.
7. Figley CR. Treating compassion fatigue. Treating compassion fatigue. London: Routledge; 2013. https://www.taylorfrancis.com/books/9780203890318.
8. Cavanagh N, Cockett G, Heinrich C, Doig L, Fiest K, Guichon JR, et al. Compassion fatigue in healthcare providers: a systematic review and meta-analysis. Nurs Ethics. 2020;27(3):639–65.
9. Klimecki O, Singer T. Empathic distress fatigue rather than compassion fatigue? Integrating findings from empathy research in psychology and social neuroscience. In: Pathological altruism. Oxford: Oxford University Press; 2012.
10. Gallese V. Embodied simulation: from neurons to phenomenal experience. Phenomenol Cogn Sci. 2005;4:23–48.
11. Zaki J. Empathy: a motivated account. Psychol Bull. 2014;140(6):1608–47.
12. Singer T, Klimecki OM. Empathy and compassion. Curr Biol. 2014;24:875–8.
13. Gilbert P. The evolution and social dynamics of compassion. Soc Personal Psychol Compass. 2015;9:239–54.
14. Jazaieri H, Jinpa GT, McGonigal K, Rosenberg EL, Finkelstein J, Simon-Thomas E, et al. Enhancing compassion: a randomized controlled trial of a compassion cultivation training program. J Happiness Stud. 2013;14(4):1113–26. http://link.springer.com/10.1007/s10902-012-9373-z.
15. Lama D, Thupten J. The power of compassion. Delhi: HarperCollins; 1995.
16. Chodron P. Tonglen, the path of transformation. Halifax: Vajradhatu Publications; 2001.

Being Mindful in a Mindless World

4

Dana Burns, Carla Nye, and Catherine Grossman

4.1 Being Mindful in a Mindless World

Healthcare professionals (HCPs) often operate in high stress environments. Efforts to achieve the Triple Aims of Healthcare [1]: improved patient experiences, reduced cost, and improved health of the population, have, in part, led to the unintended consequence of an increased prevalence of HCP burnout. The rapid and chaotic intrusion of patient, system, and personal data combined with the need to make swift and high-quality evidence-based decisions can leave HCPs feeling overwhelmed and stressed. These situational factors are correlated with increased burnout and decreased retention [2–5]. Bodenheimer and Sinsky [6] suggested adding a fourth aim to Berwick's model: improved provider experiences. The goal of this fourth aim is to identify and implement strategies that can help providers maintain or build a sense of work-life balance, while simultaneously creating environments of care that provide high quality and cost-conscious improvements to the health of our population.

As HCP's, we are pulled in many directions. At times it seems impossible to thrive when we are just struggling to survive. In our work environments, our focus is directed toward the health and safety of our patients and our co-workers. A focus on self is often a lower priority [7]. To be an effective HCP, we must shift our focus to include attention to our physical, mental, and spiritual well-being. Prior to engaging in this curriculum, HCPs may think that mindfulness is just one more task that needs to be added to an already busy day. However, this chapter will highlight the

D. Burns (✉) · C. Nye
Virginia Commonwealth University, Richmond, VA, USA
e-mail: dburns@vcu.edu; cnye@vcu.edu

C. Grossman
Pulmonary and Critical Care Medicine, Virginia Commonwealth University Health Systems, Richmond, VA, USA
e-mail: catherine.grossman@vcuhealth.org

© The Author(s), under exclusive license to Springer Nature Switzerland AG 2022   27
S. E. Braun, P. A. Kinser (eds.), *Delivering Compassionate Care*,
https://doi.org/10.1007/978-3-030-91062-4_4

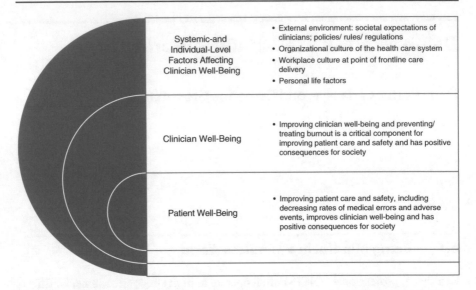

Systemic-and Individual-Level Factors Affecting Clinician Well-Being	• External environment: societal expectations of clinicians; policies/ rules/ regulations • Organizational culture of the health care system • Workplace culture at point of frontline care delivery • Personal life factors
Clinician Well-Being	• Improving clinician well-being and preventing/ treating burnout is a critical component for improving patient care and safety and has positive consequences for society
Patient Well-Being	• Improving patient care and safety, including decreasing rates of medical errors and adverse events, improves clinician well-being and has positive consequences for society

Fig. 4.1 Framework for understanding clinician well-being in the context of systemic and personal factors

complex reality of being a HCP and will introduce realistic ways to incorporate mindfulness into one's current daily routines. This will set the stage for the importance of this mindfulness curriculum for building resilience and improving retention of psychologically healthy professionals in the workforce [8–11].

Figure 4.1 provides a framework for understanding the multiple factors impacting HCPs well-being, which also impacts patient care and safety. This framework was informed by work by the National Academies of Sciences, Engineering and Medicine [12] and the National Academy of Medicine (NAM) Action Collaborative on Clinician Well-Being and Resilience [13]. The framework illustrates the myriad of mediating factors that influence our professional and personal lives. These factors include societal expectations of healthcare workers; organizational level issues within the health system; workplace culture (local workplace factors that can impact the process of performing our job); personal life factors (friendships, family matters, other community membership); and personal well-being (intrinsic to our self, maintenance of resilience, and our handling of distractions). Awareness of the multiple sources that lead to clinical burnout is key to begin the process of developing the personal and professional skills, such as mindfulness, that can assist in building well-being and resilience [14]. While this book provides a mindfulness curriculum for HCPs at the individual level, it must be acknowledged that systems level factors play a significant role in stress and burnout of HCPs [12, 13]. Mindfulness interventions are an opportunity to build resilience at the personal level. However, intentional systemic changes that support a healthy work environment are fundamental for the optimal health and well-being of HCPs [15]. For example, we assert that the integration of a curriculum such as this one into training programs for HCP students and into the offerings of healthcare systems might be one step toward larger change. In addition, protecting the time of individuals in a system to create a culture that embraces and discusses mindfulness practices may also be an important step.

4.2   Mindfulness as an Intervention for Positive Change

To enhance our ability to flourish in high demand work environments and ever evolving personal lives, HCPs can benefit from a mindfulness practice to build resilience and cultivate caring connections with self and others [16, 17]. The concept of mindfulness has been woven into Eastern cultures for thousands of years. It has been defined as "the awareness that arises from paying attention, on purpose, in the present moment and non-judgmentally" [18]. In the past, measuring mindfulness remained elusive and open to interpretation, which created barriers to systemic evaluation and utilization. In an effort to capture the essential elements of mindfulness for future research, Shapiro et al. [19] published a theoretical model that focused on the facets of mindfulness. The Intention, Attention, and Attitude (IAA) model (Fig. 4.2) identified three simplified components of mindfulness. Intention, attention, and attitude were identified, not as distinct parts, but as fluid concepts that flow together to create a state of mindfulness. Shapiro acknowledges that individual improvements in each of these facets occur in a stepwise fashion, based on individual practice. Shapiro's [20] research identified that individual practice evolves from self-regulation (regulation/acceptance of thoughts, feelings, emotions), to self-exploration (looking inward), and ultimately culminates in self-liberation

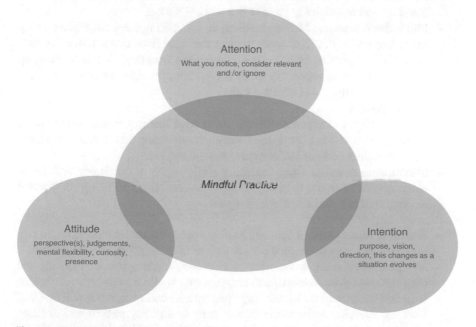

Fig. 4.2 Core components of mindfulness

(letting go, self-compassion, opportunity for growth). Intention, Attention, and Attitude will be presented as separate facets of mindfulness practice with examples from each of the authors' perspectives.

4.3 Intention: What Do You Want to Cultivate or Develop with Mindfulness? How Do You Want to Show Up for the World?

People practice mindfulness for many different reasons such as reducing stress, improving focus, increasing self-compassion, or lowering blood pressure. The **intention** component asks us to connect our mindfulness practice with our values, which can lead to a richer personal insight than the mere goal of self-improvement. The intention component asks the mindfulness practitioner to explicitly name a purpose for their engagement in practicing mindfulness. Integration and alignment with one's values (i.e., what is important to me?), intentions (i.e., what is my general goal for maintaining alignment with my values?), and actions (i.e., what specific practices can I do to stay in alignment with my values and intentions?) create a powerful foundation for growth. Furthermore, we can use our intention to shift from automatic responding and enter a place of meaningful connection with others by responding to situations with non-judgmental awareness, rather than knee-jerk reactions. The following are examples of intentions paired with relevant mindfulness practices from each author's professional life.

- Intensivist:
  - Intention/Value: Maintain authentic presence in the moment. I intend to be mentally and emotionally present in a work situation.
  - Mindfulness practice: Moving meditation, e.g., taking the stairs when coming to work to create time and space to clear the mind from one activity (being at home) before moving into another (starting the workday). While walking up the stairs, I silently repeat my goals (be present, provide medical care to the best of my abilities) as I take the stairs.
- Academic Faculty:
  - Intention/Value: Create a positive collaborative learning environment where students can flourish. I intend to model communication and interaction behaviors that reflect genuine curiosity and mutual respect.
  - Mindfulness practice: Deep breathing while saying a quick prayer prior to entering the classroom to hone and focus my intentions on being curious and respectful of my students and colleagues.
- Primary Care Practitioner:
  - Intention/Value: Create a safe and healing space. I intend to slow down to create space and time to create a deeper authentic connection with the patient.
  - Mindfulness practice: A centering ritual of handwashing to calm the body and clear the mind prior to entering the exam room. While washing my hands with soap and warm water, I silently say "just breathe and everything will be OK." I set my intention to be authentically present with my patient and to listen without judgment during this quiet moment while handwashing.

4.4   Attention: What Are You Focusing On? Where Are Your Thoughts?

The unwritten reality of healthcare is that it inherently does not follow a set schedule. We acknowledge that we work within systems that have unrelenting demands for our attention. Ad hoc events are common in healthcare, and HCPs have no control over the schedule of many parts of their work day. We are expected to be "on" a majority of our work hours. Each of these "unplanned for" events is, in essence, a distraction from other tasks, increasing our extraneous cognitive load, and taxing our mindfulness reserve as we move through the work day.

The concept of **attention** is that we maintain focus on what most requires that focus at the moment. During a mindfulness practice, it might be deliberately maintaining attention to our breath or paying attention to our surroundings in the present moment; during an interaction with a colleague, it might be maintaining focus to what they are saying without attending to the pull of distractions. The ability to stay focused is inhibited by the bombardment of internal and external data sources. Rapid triage and compartmentalization of data is required, but can lead to cognitive overload. Continuous, unremitting or poorly managed cognitive loads have been correlated with burnout [21, 22]. Focused attention can mitigate the tendency for distraction and is at the core of training mindfulness.

Focusing one's attention in the present moment and creating the space to be with one's self is the challenging work of mindfulness. In the absence of mindfulness, our attention is distracted, pulled in different directions, and scattered—we "spend" our attention without regard for how it may be affecting us and our lives. With mindfulness, we train the mind to be attentive to the intentional object of our choosing. In doing so, we decide how and on what to "spend" our attention. The ability to maintain focus on an object, one's breath, or the sensations of the present moment is a skill that can be improved with practice. Neuroplasticity research demonstrates that with repeated mindfulness meditation practice, we build and cultivate neural pathways that increase our capacity to develop a mental or physical skill [23, 24]. The purpose of honing and refining the skill of attention is not only so we can strengthen our ability to maintain this focus during, say, a meditation but also so we can maintain attention in our daily lives. As Kabat-Zinn [18] says, this is the mindful muscle that we build with consistent practice. As we become aware of what we pay attention to, we gain clarity into our inner thoughts and feelings as well as our external experiences; we are growing, evolving and expanding our ability to connect with ourselves and others.

Many actions to support attention can be incorporated into a daily routine. Examples of focusing one's attention in the workplace can include both intentionally organizing your work time to support attentive periods and maintaining attention in the present moment while in a chaotic environment. Examples of practices from the authors that help with focusing attention include:

- Intensivist:
  - Workplace challenge that threatens attention: performing clinical duties while attempting to rapidly classify the importance of information from multiple sources (i.e., personal thoughts/feelings, electronic communications, hallway conversations, alarms from devices and monitors, visual interpretation of staff and patient behaviors.)
  - Daily mindfulness practice to hone attention: open-awareness meditation to notice thoughts as they come and go in real time, practicing non-judgment when the mind gets attached to a thought, and practicing refocusing. To be able to keep our attention in the moment we must be aware of what steals our attention, know how we respond to distractions, and not judge ourselves for being distracted.
  - Honing attention in the workplace: An example of this strategy is explicitly acknowledging when distractions to attention have occurred in the workplace (e.g., ventilator alarms, pager demands, conversations amongst healthcare providers, clinical emergencies, physical disruptions of rounds), handling what is necessary, and then verbally committing to refocus on the immediate task at hand.
- Academic Faculty:
  - Workplace challenge that threatens attention: juggling competing priorities of any work day. Throughout the day, multiple shifts in attention between high and medium priority items are required. This often leaves me feeling like I am being controlled by external forces, rather than me feeling in control of my time; that I am never able to fully finish any specific work product, and I have to reprioritize every minute.
  - Honing attention in the workplace: I schedule time on the calendar to work on specific work products. During scheduled time, I turn off email and close any open windows on the computer that do not relate to the identified product. I set a timer for 25 or 50 min so that there is a clear start and end time to the work on the product. These discrete time periods give me permission to focus attention on a single product for a period of time, without feeling like other products have been neglected.
- Primary Care Practitioner:
  - Workplace challenge that threatens attention: In a short 15-min outpatient visit, I find it challenging to create ideal space and conditions to connect with the patient and their chronic and acute issues in order to provide safe, high-quality patient centered care. The juggling of the multiple aspects of a patient visit (time constraints, real-time EHR data extraction, and presenting patient concerns) can derail my attention from my intention of being present and available for the patient during our time to work.
  - Honing attention in the workplace: I find it helpful to spend several minutes at the start of my day to look ahead at my schedule, paying attention to what I anticipate to be "trigger points" that might distract me from the moment. Because I have practiced meditation in my daily life and have noticed when my attention tends to wax and wane, I am able to mindfully schedule tasks that require close attention for the early part of my day when I am most alert and attentive. This workflow creates mental space which allows focus on being authentically present and "being in the moment" with a patient.

4.5   Attitude: How Am I Talking to Myself? How Are My Thoughts, Emotions, Beliefs in This Moment Impacting the Way That I See the Work and Myself?

HCPs are, in general, ambitious high-achieving ("type A") individuals who may judge themselves harshly in the face of adversity or error, with resulting self-imposed blame and shame. Being stuck in negative self-talk can impact the next series of decisions that need to be made. We do not offer ourselves as much generosity and compassion as we would a colleague, student, or patient. Extending the same compassion to ourselves is a paradigm shift that needs to be incorporated in our professional culture. HCPs are trained to be professional in interactions, which often require them to ignore or "handle" the emotions inherent in stressful situations, but not to process them in the moment. HCPs are trained to embody the appearance of professionalism, but not historically trained to acknowledge and process the wide range of emotions that are intertwined with our work.

Mindfulness practice encourages the skill or process of using an open, curious, non-judgmental **attitude** when viewing our thoughts and mental patterns, and when interacting with the world around us. It is *how* we pay attention. It allows a shift to the mindset that one does not have to be perfect, but rather that one is human with strengths and weaknesses. For example, when engaging in a meditation practice that is focused on the breath, I might notice that my mind has strayed to the past, and that I am analyzing a conversation I had with my partner; instead of berating myself for losing attention, a non-judgmental attitude allows me to first acknowledge the distraction and then gently refocus my attention on the breath. A positive attitude of kindness, caring, and self-compassion produces a much different experience when compared to a negative self-judging critical attitude. Note that this self-compassionate, non-judgmental attitude is not about letting ourselves "off the hook"—rather, it is an important method for acknowledging all of our emotions, thoughts, and actions and bringing them to light in order to understand ourselves, rather than to blame or shame ourselves. Striving to be open, accepting, kind-hearted, compassionate, and curious are attitudes that create the lens through which we process our mindfulness journey and, ultimately, our interactions with the world. Mindfulness is the compassionate practice of focusing **our attention on our intention to shape our attitude**. Examples of how the authors incorporate mindfulness practice to focus on attitude include:

- Intensivist:
  - Workplace challenge that threatens attitude: situations that can be emotionally triggering, such as the downward health spiral or death of a patient, after which I worry whether I have thought of everything that I possibly could. It can be challenging to allow space for non-judgmental self-check after these kinds of events.

- Mindfulness Practice that incorporates attitude: I have found that "The Medical Pause" can be very helpful after a serious event or cardiac arrest. It is an opportunity to not only honor the patient being cared for but also to give space for silent reflection for the healthcare team who cared for the patient [25]. "The Medical Pause" practice allows time for HCPs to acknowledge their own feelings (including the absence of emotions) about different aspects of the event (the patient's outcome, feelings about themselves, team dynamics, etc.), to practice self-kindness by not judging themselves for the emotion they are feeling, and lastly to experience the common humanity of the situation as a member of a group [26].

- Academic Faculty:
  - Workplace challenge that threatens attitude: I occasionally find it difficult to maintain composure, focus, and positivity when entering potentially contentious meetings.
  - Mindfulness practice that incorporates attitude: I try to engage in a 3-min mindfulness meditation specific to managing conflict and difficult conversations on my meditation mobile app [27] in a healthy manner prior to going into a potentially difficult meeting. I give myself time to notice and acknowledge my current feelings of worry or fear about talking with a person with whom I have some conflict, because if I try to "stuff down" those feelings, then I might not express myself as I truly intend. Instead, I reorient myself to having an attitude of openness, a sense of curiosity about this individual. This intentional focus on having an open attitude does not deny my feelings of anger or frustration or fear, but this open attitude allows my personal core values of collaboration and respect of others to be at the forefront during the meeting.

- Primary Care Practitioner:
  - Workplace Challenge that threatens attitude: I find it sometimes difficult to maintain emotional equilibrium when confronted with some challenging patient situations, particularly patients who are belligerent or blaming.
  - Mindfulness Practice that incorporates attitude: I work hard on a daily basis to adopt the mindset of curiosity and acceptance. I do so by giving myself permission to practice humble inquiry about my patients and myself, intentionally creating a non-judgmental space for the office visit, and acknowledging my emotions. When I see a patient on my schedule with whom I have had conflict, I practice "stop-breathe-be" where I stop, take a deep breath and acknowledge the anxiety that I am currently feeling, and sit for a moment with that feeling. With my next breath, I reorient myself to the possibility that this patient might not be difficult today and/or that their belligerence might not reflect my inabilities or deficiencies. This attitudinal shift allows me to create a mutually safe space for connection, allowing crucial conversations and shared decision-making with the understanding that not all problems can be solved.

4.6   Conclusion

Healthcare professionals are struggling with the constant bombardment of data that interferes with our attention, unrealistic expectations that strain our intentions, and increased negativity that harden our attitude. Intrinsic and external forces impact our professional and personal lives. Healthcare professionals have to work hard to thrive during this complicated journey. The constantly changing and evolving dynamics cannot be solved with working harder, but with learning to slow down and "be present" with ourselves in our everyday lives. There needs to be a shift in our perspective, on an individual and systems level. Mindfulness has proven to promote positive changes in our brains, bodies, and overall well-being. The addition of mindfulness to the professional training and clinical work environments and the intentional cultivation of mindfulness in our personal lives can assist HCPs to make positive steps to create a more mindful healthcare environment in an often mindless world.

References

1. Berwick DM, Nolan TW, Whittington J. The triple aim: care, health, and cost. Health Aff (Project Hope). 2008;27(3):759–69. https://doi.org/10.1377/hlthaff.27.3.759.
2. Balch C, Freischlag J, Shanafelt T. Stress and burnout among surgeons understanding and managing the syndrome and avoiding the adverse consequences. Arch Surg. 2009;144(4):371–6. https://doi.org/10.1001/archsurg.2008.575.
3. Moss M, Good VS, Gozal D, Kleinpell R, Sessler CN. A critical care societies collaborative statement: burnout syndrome in critical care health-care professionals. A call for action. Am J Respir Crit Care Med. 2016;194(1):106–13. https://doi.org/10.1164/rccm.201604-0708ST. PMID: 27367887
4. Phillips C. Relationships between workload perception, burnout, and intent to leave among medical-surgical nurses. Int J Evid Based Healthc. 2020;18(2):265–73. https://doi.org/10.1097/XEB.0000000000000220.
5. Schlak AE, Aiken LH, Chittams J, Poghosyan L, McHugh M. Leveraging the work environment to minimize the negative impact of nurse burnout on patient outcomes. Int J Environ Res Public Health. 2021;18:1–15. https://doi.org/10.3390/ijerph18020610.
6. Bodenheimer T, Sinsky C. From triple to quadruple aim: care of the patient requires care of the provider. Ann Fam Med. 2014;12(6):573–6. https://doi.org/10.1370/afm.1713.
7. Egan H, Keyte R, McGowan K, Peters L, Lemon N, Parsons S, Meadows S, Fardy T, Singh P, Mantzios M. 'You before me': a qualitative study of health care professionals' and students' understanding and experiences of compassion in the workplace, self-compassion, self-care and health behaviors. Health Profess Educ. 2019;5(3):225–36.
8. Fendel JC, Bürkle JJ, Göritz AS. Mindfulness-based interventions to reduce burnout and stress in physicians. Acad Med. 2021;96(5):751–64. https://doi.org/10.1097/ACM.0000000000003936.
9. Kersemaekers WM, Rupprecht S, Wittmann M, Tamdjidi C, Falke P, Donders ART, Speckens AEM, Kohls N. A workplace mindfulness intervention may be associated with improved psychological well-being and productivity. A preliminary field study in a company setting. Front Psychol. 2018;9:195. https://doi.org/10.3389/fpsyg.2018.00195.

10. Mesmer-Magnus J, Manapragada A, Viswesvaran C, Allen JW. Trait mindfulness at work: a meta-analysis of the personal and professional correlates of trait mindfulness. Hum Perform. 2017;30(2/3):79–98. https://doi.org/10.1080/08959285.2017.1307842.
11. Real K, Fields-Elswick K, Bernard AC. Understanding resident performance, mindfulness, and communication in critical care rotations. J Surg Educ. 2017;74(3):503–12. https://doi.org/10.1016/j.surg.2016.11.010.
12. National Academies of Sciences, Engineering, and Medicine. Taking action against clinician burnout: a systems approach to professional well-being. Washington, DC: The National Academies Press; 2019. https://doi.org/10.17226/25521.
13. Brigham T, Barden C, Dopp AL, Hengerer A, Kaplan J, Malone B, Martin C, McHugh M, Nora LM. A journey to construct an all-encompassing conceptual model of factors affecting clinician well-being and resilience. NAM perspectives. Discussion paper. Washington, DC: National Academy of Medicine; 2018. https://doi.org/10.31478/201801b.
14. Braun SE, Kinser P, Carrico CK, Dow A. Being mindful: a long-term investigation of an interdisciplinary course in mindfulness. Glob Adv Health Med. 2019;8:1–12. https://doi.org/10.1177/21649561.
15. Perlo J, Balik B, Swensen S, Kabcenell A, Landsman J, Feeley D. IHI framework for improving joy in work. IHI white paper. Cambridge: Institute for Healthcare Improvement; 2017.
16. Burns D. Building resilience and cultivating caring in everyday practice. Poster presentation at the American Association of Nurse Practitioners. AANPConnect: an online conference experience, September–December. 2020. https://www.aanp.org/events/aanpconnect.
17. Nye C, Burns D. Capitalizing on caring: building a resilient clinican. Podium presentation at sigma/virginia nursing association annual event; 2020.
18. Kabat-Zinn J. Full catastrophe living: using the wisdom of your body and mind to face stress, pain and illness. New York: Delacorte; 1990.
19. Shapiro SL, Carlson LE, Astin JA, Freedman B. Mechanism of mindfulness. J Clin Psychol. 2006;62(3):373–86. https://doi.org/10.1002/jclp.20237.
20. Shapiro DH. Adverse effects of meditation: a preliminary investigation of long-term meditators. Int J Psychosom. 1992;39(1–4):62–7.
21. Harry E, Sinsky C, Dyrbye LN, Makowski MS, Trockel M, Tutty M, Carlasare LE, West CP, Shanafelt TD. Physician task load and the risk of burnout among US physicians in a national survey. J Comm J Qual Patient Saf. 2021;47(2):76–85. https://doi.org/10.1016/j.jcjq.2020.09.011. Epub 2020 Oct 4. PMID: 33168367.
22. Roskos SE, Fitzpatrick L, Arnetz B, Arnetz J, Shrotriya S, Hengstebeck E. Complex patients' effect on family physicians: high cognitive load and negative emotional impact. Fam Pract. 2020;38(4):454–9. https://doi.org/10.1093/fampra/cmaa137.
23. Driemeyer J, Boyke J, Gaser C, Buchel C, May A. Changes in gray matter induced by learning—revisited. PLoS One. 2008;3(7):e2669. https://doi.org/10.1371/journal.pone.0002669.
24. Voss P, Maryse T, Cisneros-Franco M, Villers-Sidani E. Dynamic brains and the changing rules of neuroplasticity: implications for learning and recovery. Front Psychol. 2017;8:1657. https://doi.org/10.3389/fpsyg.2017.01657.
25. Medical Pause. About the medical pause. 2015. https://thepause.me/2015/10/01/about-the-medical-pause/.
26. Babenko O, Mosewich AD, Lee A, Koppula S. Association of physicians' self-compassion with work engagement, exhaustion, and professional life satisfaction. Med Sci (Basel). 2019;7(2):29.
27. Difficult Conversations. In: Headspace [Mobile application software]. 2021. http://www.headspace.com/.

Part II
The Curriculum

Module 1: Introduction to Mindfulness and Compassion

5

Sarah Ellen Braun, Christina M. Luberto, and Patricia Anne Kinser

5.1 Starting the Curriculum

The start of a group-based mindfulness curriculum can set an important tone for the entire 8-week session. In order to enhance individuals' comfort with being in a group setting and sharing experiences with each other, it is helpful to provide time for getting to know each other. It does not have to be intensive, should not take the entire session, and should not involve forcing anyone to share beyond their comfort zone. Rather, it should be a fun opportunity to "break the ice" and get to know fellow group members' in a relaxed way. The following are some suggestions for ice-breakers.

> **Group Discussion: Ice Breaker**
> Idea #1: The "Simple" Ice-Breaker: Go around in a circle—introduce yourself, state something interesting about yourself, and briefly identify why you're taking this course.
> Idea #2: the "Creative Connecting" Ice-Breaker: Go around in a circle—the first person introduces themselves and states something interesting about

S. E. Braun (✉)
Department of Neurology, School of Medicine, Virginia Commonwealth University, Richmond, VA, USA
e-mail: sarah.braun@vcuhealth.org

C. M. Luberto
Department of Psychiatry, Harvard Medical School/Massachusetts General Hospital, Boston, MA, USA
e-mail: cluberto@mgh.harvard.edu

P. A. Kinser
School of Nursing, Virginia Commonwealth University, Richmond, VA, USA
e-mail: kinserpa@vcu.edu

themselves (e.g., "My name is Byron; I am a nurse on the ICU, but I went to the beach for vacation last week and was bitten on the toe by a crab"); the next person repeats the first person's name, then introduces themselves and identifies some commonality that they have with the person prior (for example, "Nice to meet you Byron. My name is Sacha; I am a respiratory therapist and I am very allergic to shellfish, so I may need you as my nurse if I accidentally eat a crab!"); and so on. This can be an easy way to help people feel that they get to know each other quickly in a low-stress manner.

Idea #3: the "Adjective + Name" Ice-Breaker: Go around in a circle and identify yourself with an adjective that starts with the first letter of your first name plus your name. Be creative! (e.g., "Spontaneous Sarah"). Then, the next person repeats the adjective + name of the first person and identifies their adjective + name ("Spontaneous Sarah, I'm Outrageous Otto"). The next person then repeats the first and second people's adjective + name and adds theirs, and so on. The first person will have to finish the process by remembering the entire circle of adjective + names. Memorizing these can be quite challenging with a large group, but group members can help each other out— and we have found that this process of helping each other ends up facilitating group cohesion quite quickly.

5.2   GETTING STARTED: Introduction to Mindfulness

Thank you all for indulging me in our ice-breaker activity. It is so helpful to get to know each other, even if just a bit, as we start on this journey together of learning about and practicing mindfulness in our personal and professional lives.

To get started, let's touch on a few guiding principles:

1. Format of Sessions: Each session, we will start with some time for centering/ becoming present to the current moment. We will follow this with discussion about key topics, which might include using some handouts/worksheets. You might want to bring a binder to keep these handouts (note to facilitators: if there are resources, providing a binder can be quite helpful and provides a sense of cohesion). After our discussions, we will engage in a formal mindfulness practice together.

2. Personal Practice: At the end of each session, I will provide you with suggestions for "homework" prior to our next session. While the concept of homework may sound less than appealing, I encourage you to see these as opportunities for practice. As we will discuss in a moment, personal mindfulness practice is essential. We will brainstorm how to create space in your life for this practice.

3. Personal Sharing during Sessions: During our sessions, I will be talking a fair amount, but I hope that you all will feel comfortable sharing your personal thoughts and experiences. We are all in this together. While I might be the

facilitator of these sessions, I do not call myself an "expert" in mindfulness. Mindfulness is a constant process, a practice. It is not a destination and there is not a finish line. We will practice together, we will wrestle with tough concepts together. I recognize that not everyone will always feel comfortable sharing in a large group setting; given this, we will occasionally break into smaller groups to talk about our thoughts and experiences. You are never required to share anything that makes you feel uncomfortable. However, I encourage you to push yourself to go outside of your comfort zone if and when you are willing to do so.

5.3 Key Concepts

5.3.1 Introduction to Stress

I think it is safe to assume that most of us in this room have made a comment at one point in their life that "I am so stressed." But, what exactly does that mean? What is stress? Is it always debilitating and negative? Can it ever be useful?

Here, we define stress as our body and mind's reaction to a challenge, demand, or threat. Stress can be positive or, we might say, manageable; sometimes referred to as eustress. Stress can also cause negative emotions and physical tension, and be difficult to manage.

In Fig. 5.1, you can see that when stress is either very low or very high, then we might have weak or ineffective performance; the exception is when a task is very simple or routine. The original research on this concept is that we need a bit of stress to be motivated and to maintain focus—this is sometimes called the "sweet spot." But, of course too much stress can be overwhelming. We have all most likely experienced this in our daily lives. We need some degree of stress to help get us out of bed in the morning, to make sure we are on time to work or our appointments, and to keep us engaged in the task-at-hand. On the left side of Fig. 5.1, a blasé attitude can cause us to make medical errors in our professional roles or forget to pay bills in our personal lives. In the middle of Fig. 5.1, a little bit of nervousness before a presentation can provide the motivation needed to practice one's talk—this bit of stress may elevate our heart rate just enough to give us the endorphin rush we need

Fig. 5.1 Relationship between stress and performance finding the "sweet spot"

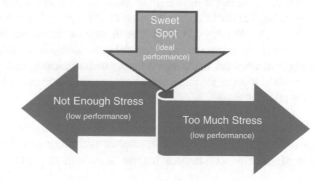

to put ourselves into an energetic "sweet spot" and give an engaging and exciting talk! However, on the right side of Fig. 5.1, a full-blown panic attack will get in the way of you being able to engage in a difficult task such as standing up in front of the audience. However, even in a full-blown panic attack, you might still be able to complete a simple task like blowing your nose or drinking a sip of water. The point is—stress can be negative or positive, depending upon various contexts and interpretations.

In other words, stress is not always a bad thing. This is why we will constantly repeat from this point forward that mindfulness is intended to help us *manage* stress, not eliminate it. The problem arises when we are overloaded by acute or chronic stressors, which not only overwhelms our psychological health but also fatigues our physical health systems, which can lead to illness as well as inability to function in our personal or professional roles. For example, we might feel repeated "negative" stress from problems at home, a high-pressure workplace, sitting in traffic, relationships, or even major weather events. This negative stress increases the biological demand on the body and causes changes in blood circulation and, if chronic or severe, can weaken the immune system. Common physical reactions of stress include high blood pressure, allergies, headaches, colds, fevers, digestive problems, memory problems, sleep changes, weight gain, concentration problems, sexual difficulties, hair loss, or skin changes. If the ability to manage stress is never addressed, these symptoms keep recurring over time.

Group Discussion
- Turn to the person next to you and tell a story about when a "positive stress" was helpful to you and when you experienced a "negative stress". What did these feel like? What did you learn about yourselves during these stories?

When there is repeated or chronic "negative stress," the physical symptoms can begin to create a change in one's attitude and beliefs about the self and others. This gives rise to unhealthy behavior changes, which can include substance use, poor sleep, overeating, unstable relationships, dissatisfaction, decreased motivation, and difficulty concentrating. Many of these are also symptoms of depression and other psychological disorders. In the case of stress, as we are discussing here, we are not referring to diagnosable disorders; though at times, stress may be comorbid with these disorders. Instead, we're referring to the cycle by which living and being in a busy and stressful world can become overwhelming and difficult to manage. It is important to separate this from psychological disorders, which have different etiologies and treatments.

As a side note, if anyone is concerned that they may be experiencing depression, anxiety, or other conditions that would warrant additional discussion, I am happy to provide references to psychotherapists and other resources in the area. Although mindfulness is certainly a helpful approach to addressing negative stress and symptoms of depression and anxiety, it is best done in combination with professional psychological help. Please note that that this curriculum is not designed to be an independent treatment for these conditions.

5.3.2 Introduction to Mindfulness

As highlighted above, stress is not always a bad thing and we will never promise that mindfulness can eradicate stress from our lives. Rather, mindfulness is an opportunity to be present to the present moment, to what is ACTUALLY going on in our lives, and to then respond appropriately to those actualities.

> **Group Activity**: watch the video by Dan Harris on "Why Mindfulness is a Superpower" (www.youtube.com/watch?v=w6T02g5hnT4). What are your reactions to this?

Let's talk about some definitions that are commonly used regarding mindfulness. Mindfulness can be defined as "paying attention to something, in a particular way, on purpose, in the present moment, non-judgmentally" [1]. Let's break this down a bit more:

- *"Pay attention to something"* this can be anything you choose to pay attention to. It often begins with paying attention to the breath but it could also be paying attention to your surroundings, driving, eating, washing dishes, your thoughts or emotions, taking a shower, your physical body, or even another person.
- *"In a particular way"* focusing on your attention, closing your eyes, and going within, looking at something, listening, tasting, smelling, or touching—with kindness, gentleness. For example, you are doing a mindfulness exercise, focusing on the breath. You notice that you lost concentration, you abruptly think of the breath, mentally kicking yourself for getting distracted, wondering to yourself why you always get distracted, there must be something wrong with you, and back to the breath, all the while kicking yourself, shaming yourself, and quickly getting distracted again. Instead, we come back to the breath (or point of focus) just as you would respond to a butterfly that landed on your arm. You wouldn't smash it or grab it. Instead can you gently, with kindness, blow it away?
- *"On purpose"* setting the intention and deciding to pay attention to this specific something.
- *"In the present moment"* means right now, while dismissing thoughts of the past or future that arise in the present.
- *"Non-judgmentally"* without assessing something as good or bad, wrong or right. It means simply perceiving with awareness and an open mind. Our tendency is to judge, and this can be useful. With mindfulness practice we learn to notice judgments, qualify them as such, and return to a nonjudgmental, open awareness state.

Other qualities or values of mindfulness include the following:

- *Beginner's mind*: approaching things as new and fresh, as if for the first time, with curiosity—even if they are something we've seen many times before.
- *Non-judgment*: impartial observation—not labeling thoughts, feelings, or sensations as good or bad, right or wrong, fair or unfair, but simply taking note of thoughts, feelings, or sensations in each moment.
- *Nonstriving*: no grasping, aversion to change, or movement away from whatever arises in the moment; not trying to get anywhere other than where you are; don't worry if this one (or any of these concepts) is confusing. And feel free to ask questions! But nonstriving especially can be difficult to understand. Think of a time when you really didn't want something to happen and it did, or a time when you really wanted something and it didn't come to be; these are examples of striving. Practicing nonstriving is a way for us to develop awareness of how our aversions (not wanting something) and desires can create suffering. It doesn't mean we can't want things or that it's bad. It is simply a reminder to notice.
- *Letting be*: simply let things be as they are, with no need to try to let go of whatever is present. Or we can keep this simple and say "open" - open to things as they are.
- *Self-reliance*: see for yourself, from your own experience, what is true or untrue. This is important. Ask questions. Remember that this is a practice of self-inquiry. You are the only one who can do it for yourself, just as I'm the only one who can do it for myself. We receive guidance from teachers and others, but it's purely experiential. Talking about it won't get us there. We've got to experience for ourselves.
- *Compassion*: cultivating love, warmth, and caring feelings for yourself and all beings, without blame or criticism. The concept of compassion and how to train it will be discussed in more depth as we move through the modules.

Group Discussion: What does "non-judgmentally" mean to you? Is that possible? What is your reaction to the phrase "self-compassion"?

How are mindfulness and well-being connected? By increasing awareness of our habitual ways of being we create the "pause" for choosing how to respond to difficult or mundane or wonderful situations as opposed to reacting out of auto-pilot.

Theoretical and empirical evidence on the effects of mindfulness training demonstrate changes in both top-down and bottom-up regulatory processes [2]. That is, meditation practice seems to allow for "a pause" in the face of stressful or emotional stimuli in which the practitioner can cognitively re-appraise stressful stimuli, thereby decreasing the resulting stress response. This top-down emotion regulation strategy is purported to be present in the early, or short-term, meditator. Long-term meditation may lead to bottom-up emotion regulation, whereby the practitioner bypasses the need for cognitive re-appraisals of stressful stimuli by decentering from thoughts and emotions through awareness that all reality arises from conscious thought. This bottom-up regulation also reduces the stress response, but more efficiently: by using less prefrontal brain connections.

Mindfulness and compassion go hand-in-hand. Compassion can be defined as the acknowledgment and desire to relieve another's suffering. With mindfulness we cultivate nonjudgmental, open awareness of the present moment. With compassion we develop the container that holds this awareness and informs our mindful quality of being. If we practice developing awareness without the container of compassion, we do ourselves a disservice. Compassion serves to transform the knowledge of our suffering and its causing into connection with others. Without the container of compassion, our mindfulness practices can show us our deepest suffering, our most ingrained habits and leave us feeling distressed and alone. With compassion, we develop a practice to transform those patterns and we learn that it is our deepest suffering that connects to others. As discussed in Chap. 3, it is important to distinguish compassion from empathy. Empathy can be thought of as the acknowledgment of another's suffering, perhaps even the desire to relieve it, but compassion transform this desire from self-focused to other-focused. Let's use an example, you are with a patient and this patient is telling you about their pain; as their clinician your job is to determine the cause of this pain and alleviate it. You feel motivated to relieve their suffering because it is your job and because you are resonating with them, as any good clinician would. Therefore, their experience of suffering is causing you distress. In this example, you are experiencing empathic distress [3]. This is a stress response in the face of another's suffering that motivates you to relieve their suffering because it hurts *you* to see them hurting. This is distinct from compassion and its motivation. With compassion, we resonate with the experience of another's suffering and we act to relieve their suffering *for them*—not to alleviate our own stress response. The result is that the compassionate clinician experiences less distress and thus less negative sequalae of stress in the face of their work. This is discussed more in Module 6 and 7.

By changing our response to stress, mindfulness and compassion practice have the ability to change the peripheral and neural substrates of stress. As HCPs working in fast-paced and high-pressure settings—often with little sleep and for long hours—this research has promising implications. The heuristics and biases the brain uses to manage the constant input of information can cause us to ignore important information, bypassing it based on past experience; with regular mindfulness and compassion practice, practitioners seem to rely less on these short-cuts and are able to process more information with less effort—even when under emotional stress. In medical practice, this could result in improved patient care and decision-making. There is a growing body of theoretical and empirical work in support of this prospect [4], and is the evidence-base for this training program [5–7].

5.3.3   Formal vs. Informal Mindfulness Practice

When we refer to the formal practice of mindfulness and compassion, we're referring to meditations in which the practitioner sets aside time, usually using a timer or recording, to practice a specific meditation. Conversely, informal practices of mindfulness and compassion are integrated into our daily life and are typically shorter.

For example, you might practice being aware of your sensations as you sit in your chair and listen to a lecture or while you're in the shower. A popular informal mindfulness technique is mindful eating. The key to informal practice is that usually other activities are going on or are only briefly paused. Throughout the following chapters, we will provide at least one formal meditation and one informal practice for each week.

Example of an Informal Practice: See the handout below for the "Stop, Breathe, Be" informal practice. We highly recommend that you try to practice this daily for the next few days, prior to our next session. We will discuss our experiences with this at that time.

How to choose formal practices? What is right for you? Take a look Fig. 5.2, the "Tree of Contemplative Practices." While not an exhaustive list of all of the possible contemplative practices out there, it can give you some ideas about some practices might help you enhance self-awareness and present moment attention. Seated

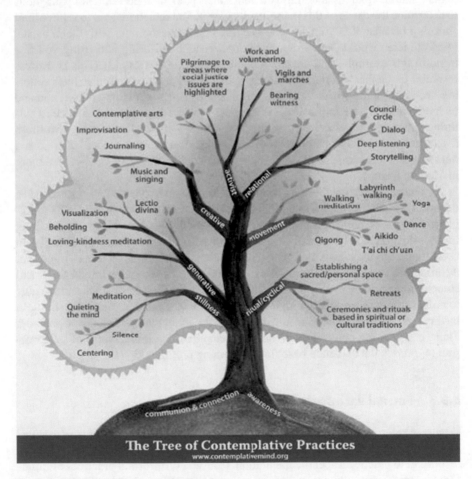

Fig. 5.2 The Tree of Contemplative Practices

meditation is not the only way to practice! Yes, there is a significant amount of research that supports meditation as an essential formal practice to learn about and build mindfulness. Throughout this manual we will focus on developing a meditation practice, but we want to encourage everyone to think "beyond the cushion" to discover other contemplative practices that you may resonate with. In fact, one can be "in the moment non-judgmentally" when being engaged in art, while chanting, even while dancing. The point is, we can bring mindful attention to anything that we do—part of your practice is to develop a toolbox for yourself of mindful and/or contemplative practices that help you be the best version of yourself. Find practices that best fit your lifestyle and your interests—and that will enhance your ability to "stick with" a regular formal practice. Check out a free yoga class near you (many studios have free classes available!); try your hand at painting or drawing; experiment with a tai chi lesson; practice guided imagery. Experiment and see what fully engages you!

5.3.4 Developing a Home Practice

Like most things in life, we only get out what we put in. This course is no different. Mindfulness and compassion can be thought of as personality traits, as states of mind, and as practices or meditations. The practice of mindfulness and compassion are crucial for the development of the traits, and the experience of them as states of mind. At first, meditating may require a lot of effort—a topic we will talk more about in the coming weeks. That is, developing a new habit can be effortful and at times we may not feel motivated or committed to the practice. If this is case for you, set a goal for yourself to practice for short periods of time, even 3 min a day is better than no minutes a day. It is important to set a goal for practice, especially in the beginning when meditation may not yet be integrated into your daily lives. Let's begin thinking about realistic goals for committing to a home practice.

[*Note to facilitators: if you will be providing or recommending specific links or resources to practices, introduce those now. Lead group discussion on setting initial goals. Attempt to guide participants to make achievable and measurable goals, encouraging daily or near-daily practice. This will continue to be a group discussion topic in the coming weeks.*]

It is also important to note that, like anything, it is not the tools themselves, but how we wield them. If we are not intentional about how we implement goals and how we talk to ourselves about meditation, we may find ourselves "guilting" ourselves into practicing meditation. Developing a new habit is a bit like walking a fine line. On the one hand, determination and diligence is required. At times, it will be difficult to stick to your goals and it may be helpful to practice even when you don't necessarily feel like it (much like waking up early for work on a cold winter's morning). On the other hand, pay attention to how you talk to yourself when you are motivating to practice or when you didn't practice but intended to. These are important moments to be gentle with yourself and remain present. When you notice that you are "shoulding on yourself", mindfulness is there, now can you invite compassion? Can you gently recommit to the practice and find the time to meditate in that moment? Or perhaps, when you notice that you are speaking harshly to yourself, can you practice Stop, Breathe, Be? This, too, is the practice. It is both the structured development of the practice—e.g., setting goals, setting timers, putting in the effort—and our *awareness of* how we talk to ourselves and *the way* we talk to ourselves when things don't go as planned.

> **Group Discussion**: What are the challenges to being mindful in your everyday life? What structures can you put into place to help you develop a daily mindfulness practice?

5.3.5   TIPS FOR INSTRUCTORS: Taking the Teacher's Seat—Who Can Instruct Mindfulness for Healthcare Professionals?

The most important experience for the facilitator of this course is their meditation practice. In that way, the teacher is no different than the student. While it is true that as teachers we must lead and guide the students, it may also be helpful to consider yourself part student. This is a practice of compassion, of not othering the students, but sitting beside them. We are *all* students of the practice. Students may ask questions about their meditation practice or about applying the qualities of mindfulness and compassion to their work, and if you, the teacher, have experience in these areas, leading and guiding becomes easy. Moreover, sharing your own experiences with meditation and integrating these qualities into your life, especially the times you fumbled or faced difficulty, can be incredibly informative for your students. This is also a practice of compassion. By showing how we've suffered—using professional self-disclosure, discussed in more detail in a later chapter—we are able to connect with others through their suffering. In fact, we recommend having a well-developed mindfulness and compassion meditation practice before endeavoring to teach this course. In the absence of this experience, teaching others would do a disservice to them and potentially lead them astray with rudimentary or misunderstood knowledge of the principles and practices. This is not a unique component of MIHP; in fact MBSR has a rigorous process that all teachers must undergo to achieve certification, which includes their own meditation practice. One year of regular meditation practice, a meditation teacher or mentor, and experience teaching or leading groups (psychotherapy, support, or college-level teaching) are our specific recommendations. That said, unlike mindfulness-based stress reduction (MBSR), there is no formal certification process for this curriculum and we encourage self-knowledge and honesty in making the decision to take the seat of the teacher.

5.4   Mindful Movement

A recommended yoga sequence to complement this chapter's theme is provided in Chap. 13.

5.5   Formal Mindfulness Practice

Note for instructors: We provide two transcripts of formal practices here, depending on how much time you have in your group session. Nevertheless, we highly recommend that the 15-min meditation be used today to initiate the group into seated meditation.

5.5.1   Focused Attention Meditation Practice: 15 min

Coming into an upright, seated posture, or if it's more comfortable for you to lay down or stand up, you may also do that. Just bringing the spine to be straight so that you're sitting or standing in an upright sort of dignified posture, but still soft and relaxed in the body. If you're sitting, you might choose to move a few inches away from the chair so that your back is self-supporting. You can let the hands rest in the lap or down at the sides, and have both feet flat on the floor. The eyes can be open, gazing down at the ground a few feet in front of you, or they can be closed.

We're going to practice a focused attention meditation. So for the next several minutes, just letting go of anything else in your day… letting everything else just fall to the sides, reminding yourself that for the duration of this practice, there is nowhere else you need to be and nothing else you need to do in these moments. Perhaps taking a breath in, breathing into a straight spine and a dignified posture, having a sense of being alert, and awake, and strong—and breathing out a sense of softening and ease, so that you're alert and awake but with a kind, easy-going attitude.

For this practice, you can choose what object of attention you'd like to focus on—you might choose the sensations of the breath, or you could choose sounds in your space. So going ahead now and setting an intention for what you're going to focus on in this practice. Choosing whichever you think will be more accessible to you today… if the breath is uncomfortable, sounds might be a nice option. If the breath comes comfortably to you, you can use the sensations of the breath. There's no right or wrong.

Whatever you choose, placing your attention there. Letting go of any expectations for what you might notice… letting go of any urges or desires to control or change the experience… just settling into an open awareness… just noticing whatever is arising moment by moment as you rest your attention on your area of focus.

[Brief pause…]

If you're using breath sensations, you might notice movement in the abdomen, the chest, or sensations of warmth or coolness at the tip of the nose. Just letting your attention rest on whichever part of the breath is most prominent for you, and just feeling the sensations as they change in that area. If you're using sounds, just letting the sounds fall to your ears. Nothing to strain or strive for, no need to even label the source of the sounds. Just resting in a receptivity, just taking in whatever you hear near and far… observing qualities like volume, pitch, or rhythm.

[Brief pause…]

At some point your attention will be drawn away from your object of focus by thoughts, distractions, anything else going on in the moment. This is part of the practice. The nature of the mind is to wander. So when you notice this happening, you can celebrate that you've noticed where your attention has gone off to; this noticing is a moment of mindfully waking up. So just noticing where the mind has gone, maybe labeling "thinking," "planning," "worrying," or whatever else, and then letting go of that and gently but firmly guiding your attention back to your object of focus. This may happen 100 times, and this just means you'll practice bringing it back 100 times. It's all part of the practice.

[1–2 min pause…]

Noticing where your attention is right now, acknowledging that, and gently coming back to your focus…

[Brief pause…]

Coming back to your focus… As best you can, just being curious about whatever you notice happening with the breath or with sounds. Can you keep your attention rested in that area to notice and explore as the experience changes moment by moment?

[Brief pause…]

If any thoughts, emotions, or sensations arise that really pull for your attention, seeing if you can be curious to explore those just for a moment, so as not to be resistant or denying that experience, but allowing yourself to see what it is just briefly… and then placing that experience to the side to gently return your attention back to wherever you're focusing.

[Brief pause…]

Noticing where the attention is right now… and getting ready to bring this practice to an end. Knowing that you've been strengthening your ability to pay attention to what you want to notice, when you want to notice it. And at any moment in your day when you notice that your mind is somewhere else, that you can celebrate that moment as a moment of mindfulness, and remember that you have the ability to guide your attention back to where you want it to be.

Perhaps inviting in some gratitude for yourself for taking time out to practice this skill. Knowing that paying attention is natural ability you always have with you, and that you're strengthening this ability each time you practice, and that you can carry this skill with you into your daily life.

You can open your eyes if they've been closed and end this practice when you're ready.

5.5.2 Mindfulness Meditation on the Breath: 5 min

To begin, you can sit comfortably and relax. It may be helpful to sit with a tall spine, without straining or overarching. You can close your eyes or leave them open with a soft focus about 3 ft in front of the tip of the nose. It's up to you. (brief pause) And now notice where the breath is most predominate. At the nostrils, at the chest, or at the abdomen. Rest your attention lightly in that area (brief pause). See if you can feel one breath from the beginning, through the middle, to the end (pause 20 s). If you're with the breath at the nostrils, you may feel tingling, vibration, warmth, coolness; at the chest or abdomen, maybe movement, pressure, stretching, release. You don't have to name these sensations, but feel them (pause 20 s). If images, or sounds, or thoughts, or sensations arise, but they're not strong enough to actually take you away from the feeling of the breath, just let them flow on by (brief pause). You don't have to follow after them, and you don't have to attack them (brief pause). You're just breathing. It's just one breath (pause 30 s). If something arises, a thought, a feeling, a sensation that is strong enough to take your awareness, your attention away from the breath, or if you fall asleep, see if you can let go and begin again (brief pause). Just bring you attention back to the breath. Even if you have to let go and begin again 1000 times, it's fine. This is the practice (brief pause). It's just one breath (pause 30 s). If you see your attention jumping to the past or the future. If you see your attention jumping toward judgment or speculation, that's okay (brief pause). Our practice is to gently let go and simply return. You keep bringing your attention back to rest on the feeling of the body breathing (brief pause). And remember, that in letting go of distraction, the important word is gentle. We gently let go (brief pause). We can forgive ourselves for having wandered and with great kindness to ourselves we begin again. Resting the awareness on the feeling of the body breathing (pause 20–30 s). And when you feel ready, you can open your eyes. Sometimes people feel more energized or exhilarated after this kind of practice, and other times they feel calm or rested, and sometimes even too rested, almost sleepy or groggy. And all of this is okay, even normal. Just see if you can bring this awareness of your breath with you as you move throughout your day.

5.6   Handouts/Resources

Stop, Breathe, Be

This is a brief exercise that you will practice this week—and you might begin to use in your everyday life. It is very simple—it is a discipline of taking a few short moments each day just to **stop** and **be** in the moment, notice what is happening, and then move on. You might want to incorporate it into your daily work by, for example, **stop**ping for a moment just before you meet with someone or go into the grocery store, take a **breath**, wait a second and allow yourself to clear your mind so that you can just **be** with the person or activity. It may seem very simple. That is ok. Some simple and obvious things can be very helpful if only we would do them!

1. **Stop.** Come to a complete and full stop. Do this deliberately. Make it full and complete. Don't move on to the next step until you have felt your body stop fully. Wait for that stop, and take long enough to feel it from the inside.

2. **Breathe**. Bring all attention to the breath. Try using either one or three breaths. Don't just notice the breath. Enter it fully, with all attention.
3. **Be**. At the end of the breath, rest in the awareness of stillness for a moment. If your eyes were closed, open them. Let any stillness or silence or relaxation that you found radiate out and saturate your environment. Allow that sense of the present moment, and its quiet center to stay with you for as long as it lasts. If it fades, don't struggle to recreate it. Instead, simply look again to see where it is. It is there already, right in that moment.

Can't remember to do this informal practice?

One idea is to put a sticker somewhere that you see regularly, as a reminder to practice "Stop, Breathe, Be"; for example, on your mobile phone or your work computer.

References

1. Kabat-Zinn J, Lipworth L, Burney R. The clinical use of mindfulness meditation for the self-regulation of chronic pain. J Behav Med. 1985;8:163–90.
2. Chiesa A, Serretti A, Jakobsen JC. Mindfulness: top-down or bottom-up emotion regulation strategy? Clin Psychol Rev. 2013;33:82–96.
3. Ekman E, Krasner M. Empathy in medicine: neuroscience, education and challenges. Med Teach. 2017;39(2):164–73.
4. Braun SESE, Kinser PAPA, Rybarczyk B. Can mindfulness in health care professionals improve patient care? An integrative review and proposed model. Transl Behav Med. 2019;9(2):187–201. http://www.ncbi.nlm.nih.gov/pubmed/29945218.
5. Braun SE, Kinser P, Carrico CK, Dow A. Being mindful: a long-term investigation of an interdisciplinary course in mindfulness. Glob Adv Health Med. 2019;8:216495611882006. http://journals.sagepub.com/doi/10.1177/2164956118820064.
6. Kinser P, Braun S, Deeb G, Carrico C, Dow A. Awareness is the first step: an interprofessional course on mindfulness & mindful-movement for healthcare professionals and students. Complement Ther Clin Pract. 2016;25:18–25. https://doi.org/10.1016/j.ctcp.2016.08.003.
7. Braun SE, Dow A, Loughan A, Mladen S, Crawford M, Rybarczyk B, Kinser, P. Mindfulness training for healthcare professional students: a waitlist controlled pilot study on psychological and work-relevant outcomes. Complement Ther Med. 2020;51:102405. https://www.sciencedirect.com/science/article/pii/S0965229919314724?casa_token=WmgnydR3JfsA-AAAA:DNGTwCmazDSLsX1DYTh7c3nj0Bw2XyK6HRkrxoYohRic2FgtOColeohgaX6oIgAtn9PDprOz0M.

Module 2: Mindfulness to Enhance Resilience and Handle Burnout

6

Patricia Anne Kinser, Chris Woods, and Sarah Ellen Braun

6.1 Key Concepts

6.1.1 Checking-In About Home Practice

As discussed previously, a consistent, personal mindfulness practice is the key to enhancing resilience in one's personal and professional life. As a facilitator of this curriculum, it is important to encourage consistent practice and to be a role model of this. Start every session with a simple formal guided mindfulness practice (see examples below). During activities, be sure to provide moments of silence for reflection and to allow for people to ask/answer questions. During wrap-up of the session, reinforce the importance of consistent practice. Review the research that is discussed in Chap. 2 about personal practice. This is a great opportunity to discuss Fig. 2.1 from Chap. 2, which highlights the differences between a stressed response and a resilient response. A resilient response is facilitated by integrating formal and informal mindfulness practices into one's life. Personal practice can be both formal and informal (see Chap. 5). Remind participants that scheduling formal practice is both necessary and important. For example, can one wake up 10 min earlier in the morning to engage in a silent meditation or yoga session? Can one block off a few

P. A. Kinser
School of Nursing, Virginia Commonwealth University, Richmond, VA, USA
e-mail: kinserpa@vcu.edu

C. Woods
Hunter Holmes McGuire Veterans Administration Medical Center, Richmond, VA, USA
e-mail: SChristopherWoods@va.gov

S. E. Braun (✉)
Department of Neurology, School of Medicine, Virginia Commonwealth University, Richmond, VA, USA
e-mail: sarah.braun@vcuhealth.org

minutes during a lunch break for a meditative walk or a short mindful breathing practice? How about trying a guided meditation right before bed?

Reminder: a consistent home practice is not easy. Just as we all experience a chattering, wandering mind, so too do we all experience the inevitable distractions that can get in the way of a formal mindfulness practice. There are unexpected impositions on one's schedule that might arise, and many of us might be tempted to put our practice to the side in order to attend to activities of the day. However, once we make a commitment to a formal practice, or at least to spending time developing these habits, then we might find that an aspect of mindful practice is learning how to put aside those distractions and impositions for a few moments.

6.1.2 Define and Discuss Burnout, Mindfulness, and Neuroplasticity

Why is a consistent mindful practice necessary? Just as building muscles in our body helps enhance strength and stability, so too does building the mindfulness muscle lend resilience during times of stress. Relevant to healthcare professionals, it is essential to discuss the concept of burnout in order to raise our awareness of the need for practices to enhance resilience against it [1].

> **Group Discussion: What Is Burnout?**
> What does it really mean to be "burnt-out"? Have you experienced this yourself or witnessed it in others?
>
> - Can you give some examples of "early signs" that you might be feeling burnt out? What thoughts, feelings, and behaviors would you see in yourself? What have you witnessed in others?
> - What are some examples of "late signs" of burnout? Have you seen these signs in yourself or in others?
> - What are the outcomes of these early or late signs of burnout, for personal and professional life?

How can mindfulness and neuroplasticity be used to enhance resilience against burnout? Let's use the following visualization.

Path in Grass Visualization:
- Close your eyes and picture a lawn of green grass.
- Now imagine that someone walks across the grass diagonally from one corner of the lawn to the opposite corner.
- Notice how the grass changes. Perhaps the grass is a bit matted down where they walked.
- Now imagine lots of people walking across the grass following the same path.
- After a while, notice that some of the grass is dying where so many footsteps have fallen.

- Imagine that this process continues until there is a path worn in the lawn where there is no longer any grass—just a dirt path worn smooth from all the foot traffic. Open your eyes.

The process of neuroplasticity in the brain is akin to a well-worn path in the grass. It is often said that "neurons that fire together, wire together." Research suggests that dendrites increase in size and efficiency when an activity, behavior, or even thought-pattern is repeated over and over [2]. Dendrites are the neuron-connectors that allow different neurons in the brain to communicate. They actually look a lot like root systems. Therefore, just like a path worn in the grass, the neuronal pathway gets stronger and stronger with repetition. Mindfulness practice is an effective way to create more healthy "pathways" in the brain [3].

Now imagine what happens to a path in grass over time when no one walks on it anymore. The grass slowly starts to grow where the path was until at some point there is no longer a path at all. Mindfulness practice can help rewire the brain so it no longer automatically responds with anxiety, or anger, or fear, or feeling stressed. Mindfulness helps adjust the pathways in the brain so that we can attend to healthy coping strategies rather than only react in anxious and fearful ways [3].

Group Discussion

- What "positive/healthy" things do you repeatedly do in your life that may have worn a "pathway" in your brain?
- What "less-helpful/less-healthy" things do you repeatedly in your life do that may have worn a "pathway" in your brain?
- Do you notice yourself responding automatically to things without stopping to think and choosing a response?
- In what ways do you feel stuck in a rut—repeating the same patterns/habits out of autopilot?

6.1.3   Mindfulness: Effortful to Effortless

Initially, when we are beginning to develop our daily practice, both the motivation to practice and the practice itself can feel effort-FULL. For example, it may be difficult to find a good time of day to practice or even to remember to practice. Likewise, when we do practice, the act of meditation may make us feel restless, bored, tired. It is important to normalize these experiences for yourself. Developing a new habit is difficult no matter the habit—an entire field within psychology is dedicated to the study and enhancement of behavior change. Also, sitting quietly and noticing the sensations of the present moment as they arise is a very unique and unprecedented activity. Most of our time is spent jumping from one stimulus to the next, seeking distractions from our screens, and being inundated with sensory information. Shifting our attention inward, with intention, is new and might cause some discomfort—this is okay. It is important to note that even after months or years of regular meditation practice, there may be days when the practice feels difficult, when the mind is restless and easily distracted or sleepy and unfocused. The art of this practice is to be aware of the present moment, no matter what. Often, mindfulness and meditation are associated with only positive attributes: calm, peace, being unburdened by thoughts, connection with nature.

> **Group Discussion**: what other positive qualities is mindfulness associated with?

Your practice of meditation will likely, at times, include those positive qualities. And, there will be moments when you encounter discomfort, pain, anger, anxiety, sadness, boredom, and an unfocused mind. How do we show up then? If we only avoid the difficult moments with distractions, then we lose the opportunity to train the mind to sit with discomforts, to become aware in the murky waters. It is this practice, this effortful training of the mind to come back to the present moment in face of suffering, that prepares us to take our practice off the cushion and into the world.

It can be helpful to think of awareness in the present moment as a target. At first, the target might be far away and very small. When we shoot our arrows of intention toward it, it requires great effort and precision to hit the target. Over time, as we develop our practice of meditation and train our mind, the target comes into focus, is within reach of our arrow, so that when we shoot our arrows of intention, it becomes almost effortless to hit the target. Many things can affect how the target appears to us on any given day, but the more we hone our mind's ability rest in the present moment, to become aware in real time, the more we are able to ride the waves from the external world and find our stillness within.

Another metaphor that may be helpful is to think of your mind as a lake. Present moment awareness lies at the bottom of the lake, the external world and all its happenings occur on the surface. The water in between are your emotions and thoughts that respond to the movement on the surface and can disrupt the ground below. Learning to identify with the bottom of the lake and not the waves above requires leaning into whatever arises and deepening awareness even when we find ourselves in difficult or stress situations.

As we move from effort-FULL to effort-LESS, we are developing a new habit and learning how to be with ourselves in times of difficulty. When practicing mindful meditation, for example, we may encounter restlessness; this is an opportunity to take a deep breath, letting it out through the mouth. We may use simple techniques like counting the breath to calm a restless mind. The tools we use serve us so that we may be present with ourselves even when the waves of life are chaotic. We then begin to take this mindful awareness with us into our lives, our work, and our relationships so that we can ride the waves of everyday life with a connection to the present moment and wider lens perspective. This connection makes it possible to respond to difficult moments instead of reacting from autopilot.

6.2   Resources/Activities

Worksheet: Identifying Your Signs of Burnout and Developing Your List of "Non-negotiables"

These lists will change over time, but it's a good idea to develop awareness of your stress and the things you need to be happy and healthy right now.

Identifying your signs of burnout:

Everyone is different and stress can show up in some strange ways. Based on your experiences thus far, what are some of the early and late warning signs that you're stressed out or burnt out? Identify physical, emotional, cognitive, and performance-based signs of stress.

1. _____
2. _____
3. _____
4. _____
5. _____
6. _____
7. _____
8. _____

Developing your list of "non-negotiables"

What are the things you need to be healthy? What are the things that become difficult to prioritize when you're overextended, but when left out of the mix make it difficult to do your job well? What are the things that "fill your cup" rather than deplete your cognitive and emotional resources? What are the practices that you do to stay at the top of your game?

1. _____
2. _____
3. _____
4. _____
5. _____
6. _____
7. _____
8. _____

6.3 Formal Mindfulness Practice

6.3.1 "Connecting Palms" Breathing Practice: 5 min

Let's sit comfortably, either cross-legged or in a chair with your feet flat on the floor. Take a few easy, long, calming breaths. If it's comfortable for you, allow your eyes to close. If that's not comfortable, let the eyes stay open with an easy focus straight ahead...

And now raise your hands up, elbows slightly bent, to the height of your heart, with your palms facing each other and hands about a foot apart. Notice how it feels to hold the arms in the air... Stay with this for a moment... Next, ever so slowly, bring the hands closer until you feel the slightest, subtle sensation of energy, pressure, heat, or warmth. Stop when you feel this... before the fingers touch. Notice for a few moments the sensation of warmth of having your palms near each other. See if you can feel the energy of the other hand, without touching.

Now bring the palms closer together until the fingertips come together with a very light touch. Imagine the energy around the molecules in the fingertips beginning to interact... Stay here for a moment... Now continue to bring the palms together until they lightly touch. As you do this, notice how the fingers straight out a bit... how more heat builds upon between your palms. This is a good time to pause for a moment, have appreciation for the body. This precious gift.

Keeping the hands where they are, spend a few moments seeing what it's like to tense and then relax the body... Keep your palms touching—now raise your elbows to the side... Press your palms together just a bit more; only 10% of the total possible pressure you could exert. Now press your hands even harder—maybe 20% of the possible pressure. Press only as hard as you can without experiencing discomfort... Still pressing at about 20% of possible effort—for a moment, observe how far up your arm the sensation of tension goes. Does it extend to wrists, elbows, shoulders, back, or chest? Do you feel more heat building up in the palms? What muscles are tense right now?

And now... let your shoulders and elbows relax and fall... release all tension completely and all at once. Let go of your hands altogether. Notice how nice it is to let go... to release tension in the body. Slowly open your palms. Sense the coolness in your palms as the heat dissipates. Let the weight of gravity tug on your hands and arms, letting them fall gently like leaves from a tree—to come rest on your lap.

Easeful breath now. Imagine stress draining out with your next exhalation... down your back, down your shoulders, your arms, your legs, out of the bottom of your feet. And let's sit for a moment in appreciation of the body, the mind, our intention, our attention, our non-judgmental attitude.

6.4 Mindful Movement Practice

A recommended yoga sequence to complement this chapter's theme is provided in Chap. 13.

6.5   Formal Meditation Practice

6.5.1   Breath Counting Meditation: 8 min

Welcome back. Today I'm going to introduce another technique for helping bring the awareness to the breath. This is called breath counting or a counting meditation. So to begin, sit comfortably with your feet on the floor, hands in your lap, close your eyes or keep them open gazing at a spot about 3 ft in front of your nose. Allow your attention to settle on the feeling of the breath, at the nostrils, the chest, or the abdomen with your normal, natural breath cycle. As you breathe in you may simply make a mental note of in and as you breathe out count one. The next breath as you breathe in you may note in and as you breathe out count two. And so on like this noting in on the inhale and counting on the exhale. So that one full in and one full out breath counts as one. Until you get to the number ten. And once you get to the number ten you return once again to one. If you become distracted and you lose touch with the breath counting before you get to ten, simply go back to one, begin again. The number, the mental noting of the number of the count is very quiet and most of the attention is on the actual feeling, the sensation of the breath. Both the note of in and the number are really a support for that awareness.

<long silence>

If you find that your attention has wandered, you needn't be upset or judgmental of yourself, just begin again at one.

<pause>

You may notice that you have thoughts or images or sensations or emotions and you're able to still keep track of the number. And if that's the case just allow those thoughts and sensations and images to come and go without getting attached to them or without condemning them.

<long silence>

You may find the rhythm of your breath changing, you may find it gets faster or slower and you can let it change as it will. Stay connected to the breath with the mental note of the number. Let the breath lead the way. Let it move, let it change as you note in one, in two, in three.

<pause>

Similarly, see if you can be with the breath as whole heartedly as possible. You don't want to say three and then be waiting for four. Just in three, in four, No matter how many times you have to begin again at one, you don't need to be discouraged. Each breath is full and complete on its own and the counting is there to support you.

<pause>

When you feel ready, you can open your eyes. See if you can bring some of this awareness with you as you move throughout your day.

6.6   Tips for Instructors

Wondering how to manage group dynamics during discussions about mindfulness? What we've found to be most helpful is to weave the exploration of dynamics into the actual process of mindful inquiry itself. It quickly becomes clear as to how different group members go about trying to deal with such things as discomfort, ambiguity, and the need for attention, etc. For example, you might notice you have a member who is a "twiddler" (a bunch of nervous energy, fidgeting and moving all about, not able to sit still) or a "rationalizer" (someone who has very clear excuses for behaviors, or who wants to exert logic/reason at all times) or a "controller" (someone who likes to lead and tries to take over the group and assume control). Don't criticize, judge, or argue with the member about these behaviors. That will take the group off course.

Instead get curious about the function (not the form) of these behaviors and now make them the focus of mindful inquiry. Gently, curiously, nonjudgmentally ask questions such as: "I just noticed you started asking a lot of questions. Is that what you do when you're feeling unsure?" With any behavior, notice it, validate it, and then explore what that behavior might be hoping to achieve (decrease in anxiety?) and then gently try to bring the focus back to the topic at hand. Just like meditation!

This can be difficult to do and if it becomes a bigger issue, it can help to share your own experience and reaction to what's happening in the room. For example, "I notice it seems like we're stuck here, or that there's some resistance. Does anyone else notice that?" At the very least, you're helping move mindful awareness along even during difficult or stuck interactions. Modeling mindful responses to situations is a key component of your role in leading this curriculum.

References

1. Maslach C, Jackson SE, Leiter MP. Maslach burnout inventory. In: Evaluating stress a book of resources. 3rd ed. Lanham: Scarecrow Press; 1997. p. 191–218. http://search.ebscohost.com/login.aspx?direct=true&db=psyh&AN=1997-09146-011&lang=fr&site=ehost-live.
2. Cramer SC, Sur M, Dobkin BH, O'Brien C, Sanger TD, Trojanowski JQ, et al. Harnessing neuroplasticity for clinical applications. Brain. 2011;134(6):1591–609. https://academic.oup.com/brain/article/134/6/1591/369496.
3. Vago DR, Silbersweig DA. Self-awareness, self-regulation, and self-transcendence (S-ART): a framework for understanding the neurobiological mechanisms of mindfulness. Front Hum Neurosci. 2012;6:1–30.

Module 3: Applications of Mindfulness as a Healthcare Professional

7

Mariah Sullivan, Jennifer Huberty, and Sarah Ellen Braun

7.1 Key Concepts

In this module, key concepts to be discussed include goal-setting regarding mindfulness practice and how one might teach mindfulness to others, such as one's patients. For each concept, we provide ways to apply this information to your personal life and to your patients.

7.1.1 Goal-Setting

You have learned what it is to have a mindfulness practice and the benefits from such a practice. But how do you go from wanting to have a mindfulness practice to actually having a mindfulness practice? Setting goals can help guide you through your journey and keep you focused on being consistent with your practice. We will use process and outcome goals [1]:

- *A process goal* is something you can control such as meditating for 10 min per day or going on nature walks three times per week. Process goals represent the steps you will take to attain the long-term outcome goal. Process goals are specific and measurable.

M. Sullivan
College of Health Solutions, Arizona State University, Tempe, AZ, USA
e-mail: msulli27@asu.edu

J. Huberty (✉)
Calm, San Francisco, CA, USA
e-mail: jen@calm.com

S. E. Braun
Department of Neurology, School of Medicine, Virginia Commonwealth University, Richmond, VA, USA
e-mail: sarah.braun@vcuhealth.org

- *Outcomes goals* represent the overall outcome you wish to accomplish by participating in mindfulness, for example, being more patient and having less stress.

The process goals will likely facilitate the outcome goals even if there is not a clear definition of what these outcome goals are. The key is in the process.

When deciding on a process goal to achieve an outcome goal, it is important to ask yourself a number of questions. First, what are your motivators (i.e., benefits) for participating in your process goal? Why do you want to do this? Second, what are some barriers that might keep you from achieving a process goal? For example, meditating for 10 min per day might be challenging when kids need to be dropped at school or your work schedule is demanding. Facilitators, on the other hand, help you overcome barriers to reach your goal. Some examples of facilitators include scheduling a time to meditate daily (you are more likely to make it a habit when you do something at the same time every day) [2], setting reminders, making a special space for your practice, and asking someone to keep you accountable. Supportive friends/relatives/communities can also help support you in achieving your process goals. What supports do you have to help you be successful at maintaining a mindfulness practice? Research suggests that you are more likely to be successful at achieving goals if your perceived benefits outweigh your perceived barriers [3]. In other words, if you believe that there are benefits to meditating for 10 min you are more likely to schedule time in your day to meditate or ask someone to remind you to meditate.

We can become more mindful if we practice mindfulness. But first, we have to be compassionate to ourselves and set ourselves up for success with strategies like goal-setting. Using known strategies, tools, and resources to practice mindfulness (process goals) is key to becoming more mindful (outcome goal).

> **Group Discussion**
> Brainstorm a few specific process goals that might help you with an outcome goal of becoming more mindful in one's daily life.

7.1.1.1 How Do I Apply This Information to My Patients?

In order to teach our patients to be mindful, we must have a mindfulness practice, ourselves. Setting and achieving our goals will help us to talk to our patients about appropriate process goals to achieve a mindfulness practice. For example, when you are meditating 10 min daily and using facilitators to help you achieve this process goal, you will understand what it took to stay committed and achieve your goals thus better able to teach your patients. Try using the worksheet at the end of this module to help you (and your patients) set and reach mindfulness goals.

7.1.2   Daily Routines

7.1.2.1   How Can Routines Help Build More Mindful, Compassionate Lives?

A daily routine is a collection of habits you do every day. Successful scientists, artists, and CEOs, such as Benjamin Franklin, Ernest Hemingway, Arianna Huffington, and Steve Jobs, are known to have daily routines to help them succeed. Routines allow us to turn the behaviors we want to perform, such as a mindfulness practice, into habits: something we do automatically without thinking about it.

Habits are formed using a four stage process: cue → craving → response → reward [4]. For example, if your goal is to meditate, you wake up and see the meditation space set up on the floor, which is your *cue*. You want to feel more peaceful and focused through the day, your *craving*. You then choose to sit and meditate for 10 min, a *response* to wanting to feel more peaceful and focused. Your *reward* is feeling this way and together, these four stages create a feedback loop that helps you create the automatic habit of meditating immediately after waking up.

Research has shown that some ways to incorporate these habits are to make them easy and rewarding [5]. To make your habit easy, the cue should be obvious and the habit should not be too demanding. For example, using a cue of a meditation space on the floor of your bedroom and meditating for 10 min are much easier than having to remember on your own (i.e., without a cue) or meditating for an hour during your already busy morning. The habit should also be rewarding. You want to meditate because you want to feel peaceful and you obtain that feeling once you've finished your practice. Maybe you would feel more peaceful by going for a walk in nature. Whatever you choose, make sure it makes you feel the way you want to feel. While some people may want to start their day by feeling peaceful and focused, others may crave this feeling toward the end of the day, wanting to wind down. There is no right or wrong time to incorporate a new habit or routine, but consider when works best for you.

Morning routines can set the tone of the day. This applies to everything you do in the morning, starting from the moment you wake up. Research suggests that morning routines can impact our mood and productivity [6]. Habits such as exposure to sunlight or exercise in the morning may help improve your circadian rhythm and help provide more energy during the day [7]. Here are some mindfulness practices that you might consider as part of a morning routine:

- Having a beverage, like water with lemon or tea, while sitting in silence.
- 10-min walk in nature or around your neighborhood.
- Sitting and breathing for 5 min.
- Listening to a guided meditation.
- Journaling.
- Reading a chapter from your favorite book.

- Yoga—sun salutations (see examples of this practice in Chap. 13).
- Exercise.
- 10 min of sunlight (sitting outside or face the sun from the indoors).
- Write and/or recite affirmations.

Evening routines are a great way to "let go" of the day. They allow you to wind down and prepare for sleep. Stress, screen usage, and other factors can interfere with the quality of our sleep so it's important to cultivate an evening routine to allow us to reach a state of deep sleep. Deep sleep is essential for mental and physical health, such as our ability to learn and our body's ability to recover [8]. For healthcare providers, sleep is especially important to prevent burnout and compassion fatigue, allowing you to provide the best possible care for patients [9]. Some habits have been suggested by research to help us prepare for sleep. For example, avoiding screens before bed allows the brain to produce melatonin, a hormone essential for regulating the sleep-wake cycle [10]. Journaling and preparing for the next day can help alleviate stress levels by allowing you to process the past and plan for the future.

Here are some mindfulness practices that you might consider as part of an evening routine:

- Journaling.
- Listening to relaxing music.
- Unplugging from electronics—leaving your phone in another room, turning off the TV.
- Going to bed at the same time.
- Reading.
- Yoga nidra.
- Create a "closing ritual" from your workday, such as tidying your desk or creating a to-do list for the next day.
- Prepare for tomorrow—choose the outfit you'll wear to work, pack your lunch, or write down tasks you need to prioritize.

Sometimes, daily routines do not go as planned. Even the most successful people who rave about their daily routines have off days, and you likely will too. That is ok! Getting off track is a perfect time to practice self-compassion: forgive yourself for not being perfect. Committing to your routine the following day, finding a routine that works better for you, and finding ways to hold yourself accountable are also part of self-compassion. The goal of daily routines, after all, is to help you create a more mindful, compassionate life. Try finding an accountability partner, such as a partner or friend, who will check in with you or, even better, has a routine of their own they are trying to uphold. Many people use a habit tracker where they check off the habits they complete each day. This can be done on paper or through various habit tracker apps.

Group Discussion
Identify one morning routine and/or one evening routine with which you have experimented in the past. How did it go? Do you continue to use that routine?
    What else would you like to incorporate into your daily life? What specific plans can you put into place to make this happen?

7.1.3   How Do I Apply This Information to My Patients?

Helping patients establish morning and/or evening routines can improve their overall health in various ways, such as practicing mindfulness or incorporating healthier food choices. Sharing the morning and evening routines that you use to be mindful may help inspire your patients to do the same. Ask your patients to begin one or two routines in the morning or evening in order to help them to start practicing mindfulness.

7.1.3.1 Tips for Instructors
We can only teach what we know. By incorporating mindfulness practices into your daily life, you will be much better able to help your patients practice mindfulness.

7.2   Resources/Activities

7.2.1   Handout

Daily Routines to Build Mindful Lives
A daily routine is a collection of habits you do every day. One reason routines can help us reach our mindfulness goals is because we are turning these new behaviors into habits, meaning we don't even have to think about them.
    Ideas for mindfulness practices that you might consider as part of a morning routine:

- Having a beverage, like water with lemon or tea, while sitting in silence.
- 10-min walk in nature or around your neighborhood.
- Sitting and breathing for 5 min.
- Listening to a guided meditation.
- Journaling.
- Reading a chapter from your favorite book.
- Yoga—sun salutations (see chap. 13).
- Exercise.

- 10 min of sunlight (sitting outside or face the sun from the indoors).
- Write and/or recite affirmations.

Ideas for mindfulness practices that you might consider as part of an evening routine:

- Journaling.
- Listening to relaxing music.
- Unplugging from electronics—leaving your phone in another room, turning off the TV.
- Going to bed at the same time.
- Reading.
- Yoga nidra.
- Create a "closing ritual" from your workday, such as tidying your desk or creating a to-do list for the next day.
- Prepare for tomorrow—choose the outfit you'll wear to work, pack your lunch, or write down tasks you need to prioritize.

Need a little help maintaining your routine? Have an "off-day" and forget to practice?

- Practice self-compassion: Forgive yourself for not being perfect. Remember that committing to your routine the following day, finding a routine that works better for you, and finding ways to hold yourself accountable are part of self-compassion. The goal of daily routines, after all, is to help you create a more mindful, compassionate life.
- Create structure: Try finding an accountability partner, a friend or family member, who will check in with you or, even better, has a routine of their own they are trying to uphold. Many people use a habit tracker where they check off the habits they complete each day, such as on a calendar or with a habit tracker app.

7.3   Worksheet

Goal-Setting for Mindfulness

Instructions: Use this worksheet to develop your goals related to an area in your life that you would like to improve or enhance.

Step 1: Choose from one of the following "life areas" that you would like to focus on right now, that might benefit from enhancing mindfulness:

- Physical health.
- Emotional health.
- Relationship.
- Friendship.
- Financial.
- Daily joy.
- Career.

Step 2—personal values: Your personal values are what you believe to be important in your life, what shapes your daily life. Think of personal values as your "compass" for helping you make decisions and goals in your life. Below are examples of values. Circle the words that matter most to you and which inform your decision-making about setting goals for mindfulness in your life.

• Trust	• Appreciation	• Openness
• Patience	• Gratitude	• Caring
• Respect	• Patience	• Compassion
• Generosity	• Peace	• Honesty
• Hospitality	• Kindness	• Humor
• Transparency	• Harmony	• Cooperation
• Attentive	• Hopefulness	• Joyfulness
• Supportive	• Service	• Calmness
• Acceptance	• Nurturing	• Understanding
• Self-acceptance	• Altruism	• Spirituality
• Curiosity	• Sensitivity	• Encouraging
• Empathy	• Faithfulness	• Thoughtfulness
• Humility	• Expressive	• Gracious
• Compromising	• Grateful	• Fairness
• Friendliness	• Sharing	• Love
• Loyalty	• Persistence	• Reliability

Step 3—Goal-Setting: Develop one process goal and one outcome goal related to enhancing mindfulness in your life, building upon what you identified as the area in your life you would like to improve and your personal values. Remember that an outcome goal is the overall outcome you wish to accomplish; a process goal is something very specific and measurable that you can control.

For example:

Outcome Goal—By enhancing mindfulness in my life, I wish to enhance my sense of gratitude and appreciation for those with whom I have a personal relationship.

Process Goal—Every evening, I will spend 5 min on a guided meditation on my mindfulness app that relates to gratitude.

7.4 Mindful Movement Practice

A recommended yoga sequence to complement this chapter's theme is provided in Chap. 13.

7.5 Formal Meditation Practice

7.5.1 How to Talk to Yourself Meditation: 6 min

Welcome back. Today we will be paying particular attention to the moment when we realize we're distracted and how we speak to ourselves. We say that the moment you realize you've been distracted is this magic moment because that's the moment that we have the chance to be really different: to respond differently, to relate differently to ourselves, to not judge ourselves, not condemn ourselves, but to simply let it go and begin again. So, sit comfortably, close your eyes or not, and then allow your awareness to settle on the place where the breath is the most predominant at the nostrils, chest, or abdomen. And bring your attention to that area to just rest. Feel one breath at a time.

<long silence>

If something arises, sensations, images, fantasies, memories, planning, motions, whatever it might be that's strong enough to take your attention away from the feeling of the breath, notice how you speak to yourself as you prepare to let go and begin again. If it's in a harsh, judgmental voice, see if you can soften. It is actually with kindness toward ourselves, rather than condemning ourselves, that we make the most progress. It doesn't matter how many times your attention wanders or how long you dwell in a particular distraction. It also doesn't matter where your attention wandered to. The goal is the same, let go gently and with growing kindness toward ourselves, we begin again.

<long silence>

When you notice that your mind has lost its awareness on the breath and gotten carried down a rabbit hole, that's ok! Let it go and gently, with kindness, come back to rest the awareness and the feeling of the body breathing. And when you're ready you can open your eyes. So this moment after we notice that we have wandered, that we've been distracted, this is a crucial moment when we practice letting go and beginning again. And this is the art of the practice. So see if you can bring some awareness of kindness toward yourself throughout your day, perhaps even noticing how you speak to yourself. Noticing if it's different how you to speak to yourself when you're at home or when you're at work. Or see which times of day you find it the easiest and most challenging to be kind to yourself.

References

1. Zimmerman BJ, Kitsantas A. Developmental phases in self-regulation: shifting from process goals to outcome goals. J Educ Psychol. 1997;89(1):29.
2. Wood W, Quinn JM, Kashy DA. Habits in everyday life: thought, emotion, and action. J Pers Soc Psychol. 2002;83(6):1281.
3. Sieber SD. Toward a theory of role accumulation. Am Sociol Rev. 1974;39(4):567–78.
4. Clear J. Atomic habits: tiny changes, remarkable results: an easy & proven way to build good habits & break bad ones. New York: Avery; 2018.
5. McCloskey K, Johnson BT. Habits, quick and easy: perceived complexity moderates the associations of contextual stability and rewards with behavioral automaticity. Front Psychol. 2019;10:1556.
6. McClean ST, Koopman J, Yim J, Klotz AC. Stumbling out of the gate: the energy-based implications of morning routine disruption. Pers Psychol. 2021;74(3):411–48.
7. Yoon IY, Song BG. Role of morning melatonin administration and attenuation of sunlight exposure in improving adaptation of night-shift workers. Chronobiol Int. 2002;19(5):903–13.
8. Samson DR, Nunn CL. Sleep intensity and the evolution of human cognition. Evol Anthropol. 2015;24(6):225–37.
9. Åkerstedt T, Kecklund G, Axelsson J. Impaired sleep after bedtime stress and worries. Biol Psychol. 2007;76(3):170–3.
10. Fossum IN, Nordnes LT, Storemark SS, Bjorvatn B, Pallesen S. The association between use of electronic media in bed before going to sleep and insomnia symptoms, daytime sleepiness, morningness, and chronotype. Behav Sleep Med. 2014;12(5):343–57.

Module 4: Interpersonal Mindfulness and Compassionate Patient Care

8

Jennifer Huberty, Mariah Sullivan, and Mindy Loiselle

8.1 Key Concepts

In this module, key concepts to be discussed include awareness of automatic thoughts and compassionate listening. For each concept, we provide ways to apply this information to your personal life and to your patients.

> **Group Discussion:**
> In the previous module, you developed a personal process and outcome goals regarding mindfulness practice.
> Have you been able to follow through on your process goal? How is it going for you?
> If it is not going as you had hoped, what modifications might you consider regarding the goal itself and/or structuring your time in order to meet your goals?

8.1.1 Awareness of Automatic Thoughts

Daily routines can put us in the right frame of mind to be more mindful throughout the day, a key part of which is noticing our thoughts.

J. Huberty (✉)
Calm, San Francisco, CA, USA
e-mail: jen@calm.com

M. Sullivan
College of Health Solutions, Arizona State University, Tempe, AZ, USA
e-mail: msulli27@asu.edu

M. Loiselle
Psychotherapist/ Licensed Clinical Social Worker, Richmond, VA, USA

© The Author(s), under exclusive license to Springer Nature Switzerland AG 2022
S. E. Braun, P. A. Kinser (eds.), *Delivering Compassionate Care*,
https://doi.org/10.1007/978-3-030-91062-4_8

We have about 6000 thoughts per day [1], but our minds are only in the present moment for about 3 s at a time. Otherwise, we are thinking in either the past or the future often without realizing it. Think about how many times, even while reading this chapter, your mind went somewhere else: items on your to-do list you will tackle next, the conversation you had at work yesterday, what you will eat for dinner. Our minds wander in ways we don't necessarily choose and we are oftentimes not even aware that this is happening.

Automatic thoughts usually reflect patterns of thinking that we have established over the years, and they are typically negative or reactive. For example, maybe whenever someone gives you a compliment your first response is to think, "Oh, she's just saying that to be nice. She doesn't really mean it." Perhaps whenever you make a mistake, your first response is to blame yourself or someone else, to become angry or frustrated, or to feel hopeless about correcting the problem. Each of these is an automatic thought and oftentimes not true or helpful. However, as with any thoughts we have, we cannot change them until we become aware of them.

Noticing thoughts becomes easier as we establish a mindfulness practice. Sitting in silence for at least 5–10 mins daily, tuning into our senses, will help you become more aware of your thoughts in the long term. But at first you just want to try to notice your thoughts during the day. You may find that you are harder on yourself than you thought or maybe you have a more negative view about life that you want to have. The first step is to just notice the thought, without judgment. Once we are able to begin to become aware of our thoughts we can start to question and challenge them. For example, if the first thought that comes to mind after making a mistake is, "I'm horrible at this." Ask yourself, Is that true? Can I find a new perspective? You might realize that you have countless other talents and your one mistake doesn't determine your value or skill level. Finally, we can try to introduce compassion into the situation. Would you say this negative thought about yourself to your best friend or family member? We can show ourselves the same amount of compassion as we have for those we love. You might imagine you are talking to someone you love after they made a mistake. What might you say instead?

8.1.2   How Do I Apply this Information to My Patients?

As you become better at being aware of your thoughts, you will notice how your thoughts contribute to your practice as a provider. You will be able to be less judgmental of yourself and more compassionate, which means it will be easier to do the same with your patients. It will also help you to be a more present listener which we will discuss next.

8.1.3   Compassionate Listening

Do your best to practice compassionate listening. Do not listen for the sole purpose of judging, criticizing or analyzing. Listen only to help the other person express himself and find some relief from suffering. -- Thich Nhat Hanh

Compassion is the capacity to acknowledge and have sympathy to someone else's suffering or misfortunes [2]. Compassionate listening implies being present and listening attentively in the moment. Compassionate listening brings humanness, patience, and vulnerability to interacting with another human in a meaningful way, potentially alleviating some of his or her suffering. Compassionate listening allows others to be themselves without any worry about disapproval. There are certain skills that are required to be a compassionate listener and may include emotional strength, patience, openness, and a desire to understand someone else's feelings [3]. Some practices for compassionate listening include (1) Direct participation—Look at a person directly and pay attention to body language, (2) Show interest—Focus on what the person is saying without thinking about a reply, (3) Check-in on your body language and make sure it is open and inviting, (4) Make eye contact, (5) Listen without judgment—listen without interrupting or making suggestions, (6) Take deep breaths—breathing will help keep you calm without losing focus.

Next time you talk to someone, whether a friend, family member, or patient, notice your ability to listen compassionately. Are you making eye contact and truly being present or are you multitasking? Does the speaker know you are interested in what he or she has to say? Are you able to summarize and repeat what the speaker just said or were there parts where you zoned out? Practicing this skill can improve all of our relationships by improving our communication and conveying the message that we care about the other person.

Group Activity: Active Listening

Being attentive and present is important when interacting with others, whether in your personal or professional life. One way to practice truly listening is to engage in this "active listening" practice. You may have heard of this before. The speaker tells any story they would like (today- how about telling a story about a stressful situation, how you handled it, and what you learned about yourself). The challenge is for the listener to be completely open—you should JUST listen. Don't talk or respond in any way. Try to even avoid using physical cues such as nodding or smiling. Practice being totally open to the speaker, without trying to think of what you could say in response to their story. This is an opportunity to create space for the speaker's experience.

Ready? Pair up now. One person is the speaker for 5 mins, one is the listener. After 5 mins, I will tell you that time is up and to switch roles.

Group Discussion:

How did it feel to be the "active listener"? How did it feel to be the speaker? Reflect upon how you can use elements of this experience in your daily life.

8.1.4   How Do I Apply this Information to my Patients?

One of the most common complaints about providers from patients is that patients feel that their providers don't listen to them. Providers are busy; they see numerous patients and have limited time with each patient. A mindfulness practice will help you to be more present and aware with the limited time you have, which means you will be aware of your thoughts and a more active, compassionate listener. As an active listener, you will create space for your patients to share their experiences. Overall you and your patients are likely to be more satisfied with the time spent.

8.2   Tips for Instructors

Compassionate listening is a skill that takes practice, but you can help your students develop this skill by modeling compassionate listening. They will likely notice how they feel after a conversation with you and want to emulate your compassionate listening skills with others.

8.3   Handout

21 Ways to Practice Mindfulness

Below is a list of ways that you can practice mindfulness; feel free to share this with your patients.

1. Listen to guided meditation (mobile apps, YouTube, Spotify, Calm, etc).
2. Close eyes and tune into sounds and breath (unguided meditation).
3. Yoga (personal practice, classes, mobile apps, Udaya.com).
4. Reading your favorite book.
5. Drawing/painting/ Mindful coloring.
6. Breathing exercises (mobile apps have many examples of these).
7. Journaling—writing.
8. Walking in nature—spending time outside.
9. Gratitude—send a card to someone.
10. Appreciation lists.
11. Planting/gardening.
12. Engaging with animals (e.g., petting a dog or cat, watching hummingbirds).
13. Mindful eating—slow chewing, tasting.
14. One task at a time (withdraw from multitasking).
15. Feel your feelings—awareness of your emotions—observation of emotions.
16. Engage in your favorite hobby (e.g., baking, scrap books).
17. Physical activity that is mindful—requires attention—(e.g., Tai Chi, yoga).
18. Mindful showering/body care—paying attention to temperature, your skin.
19. Listen to your favorite song or calming music.
20. Tune into your senses—smelling lotions/oils, scents.
21. Disengage with social media and tune into what is going on around you.

8.4   Mindful Movement Practice

A recommended yoga sequence to complement this chapter's theme is provided in Chap. 13.

8.5   Formal Meditation Practice- Two Options

8.5.1   Option 1: Gratitude Meditation

Sit in a comfortable position that allows your back to be straight, perhaps on a cushion or chair. Start to tune into your body and the space around you. Notice the parts of your body that are touching the cushion or chair. Relax your shoulders and neck. Relax your face. Notice the natural rhythm of your breath. Inhale. Exhale. Without trying to judge or change anything, just notice each breath. Your breath might start naturally slowing down as you start to relax. Feel your muscles slowly relaxing and continue to breathe.

[long pause]

Now begin to think about things you are grateful for. Those you love, nature, a certain color, your health, safety—whatever makes you feel grateful. Think about those things, one at a time, and express your gratitude. Maybe you say thank you, maybe you smile, maybe you extend a warm hug. Continue to spend time with each "thing" you are grateful for and bask in the gratitude.

[long pause]

Notice how you are feeling. Allow this feeling of gratitude to move up and down your body and all around you. Enjoy the feeling of joy and appreciation. You can continue this mediation as long as you like. You might find that as you become more filled with gratitude and joy your list gets longer and longer. When you are finished with your meditation, pause for a moment, start to come back to the place in which you are sitting, the room you are in, the noises and sensations around you. Now bring this feeling of gratitude with you during your day.

8.5.2   Option 2: Compassionate Heart Meditation

Come into a comfortable seated position. Let your eyes be open or closed, whatever is comfortable for you. Set a desire or intention: the longing to ease suffering by cultivating your compassionate heart.

Take a long breath in through your nose and release it in a long slow exhale through pursed lips like you are blowing out through a straw. Breath in this manner a few more times.

Return to your natural breath. Know that you are breathing.

Notice your desire that all beings be free from suffering. Remind yourself of your compassionate heart. Feel your heart space. Notice whatever is present.

Be aware of the signals from your body and mind. Be present to what is and respond; breathe, remind yourself of your intent to cultivate compassion. Reactions are conditioned responses-no need for judgment, rejection. Pause. Breathe.

Notice your body. Breath in and out. Create space for what is. Is there closing? Is there contraction? Is there openness? Is there space? Greet what is with spacious compassion. Kind, open, patient, tolerant.

Remind yourself of your own compassionate heart. Compassion for one-self...compassion for others. Receive what is without evaluation. Remind yourself of your intent and desire to relieve pain and suffering in oneself and others.

Breath in care and compassion for all beings; breath out care and compassion for all beings.

Bring your meditation to a close by gently opening your eyes if closed and notice your surroundings. Thank yourself for meditating.

References

1. Tseng J, Poppenk J. Brain meta-state transitions demarcate thoughts across task contexts exposing the mental noise of trait neuroticism. Nat Commun. 2020;11(1):1–12.
2. Kimble P, Bamford-Wade A. The journey of discovering compassionate listening. J Holist Nurs. 2013;31(4):285–90.
3. Zahed DH. (2017, July 11). Compassionate listening. HuffPost. Retrieved October 26, 2021, from https://www.huffpost.com/entry/compassionate-listening_b_10921036.

Module 5: Mindful Teams and Leadership

9

Alisha Gupta and Christopher S. Reina

9.1 Key Concepts

9.1.1 Team Functioning

Given the complexity of delivering healthcare, healthcare typically operates in the form of interdisciplinary teams when caring for patients. For example, physicians, nurses, and others collaborate, with the shared common goal of high-quality patient care. It is thus important for us to understand how teams function in order to effectively carry out our tasks as healthcare professionals [1]. In this chapter we emphasize the importance of understanding how we "show up" and engage with each other on the healthcare team, requiring awareness of one's thoughts and emotions when they come to work and engage with others. Remember, also, that developing mindfulness as a leader is essential because the leader impacts effectiveness of the healthcare team [1–4].

9.1.2 Reviewing the Definition of Mindfulness

As we have been discussing throughout this curriculum, we can think of mindfulness as a nonjudgmental way of paying attention to particular thoughts, feelings, and emotions [5, 6]. We refer to mindfulness as sustained attention to the present moment (rather than the past or future) and being aware of thoughts and emotions as they occur [7–9]. In other words, mindfulness involves intentionally paying attention to the present moment with less judgment and self-focus. Researchers have found that consistent mindfulness practice can influence individuals' emotional well-being [10–13], self-regulation and rumination [11], stress [14], emotional exhaustion [15], and even motivation and performance across the workweek [16].

A. Gupta · C. S. Reina (✉)
Virginia Commonwealth University School of Business, Richmond, VA, USA
e-mail: guptaa26@vcu.edu; csreina@vcu.edu

© The Author(s), under exclusive license to Springer Nature Switzerland AG 2022
S. E. Braun, P. A. Kinser (eds.), *Delivering Compassionate Care*,
https://doi.org/10.1007/978-3-030-91062-4_9

Consider the current challenges to clinicians who are overlaid with back-to-back patient appointments and pressured to chart each interaction in increasingly advanced electronic medical records. It is not uncommon for clinicians to get caught up on the computer while simultaneously trying to listen to patients' concerns. Training mindfulness can enhance how clinicians engage with patients, especially in the current climate of demanding schedules.

9.1.3 Mindful Leadership

Mindfulness has important benefits for all of us no matter our position, but it may be especially helpful for effective leadership. First, research shows that mindfulness can improve self-leadership capacities such as task management, self-care, and self-reflection [17–19]. Second, researchers are beginning to explore how a leader's mindfulness may help them enact more justice while reducing stress and exhaustion for their employees as well as increasing employee performance and well-being [20–23].

Important to our work as leaders in healthcare, leader mindfulness has been linked with the ability to relate to others via increased listening quality, awareness of followers' needs, decreased emotional reactivity, as well as less judgment and self-involvement [19].

> **Group Discussion: How Might Mindfulness Benefit Leaders?**
> Consider a typical 12-hour nurse shift. Nurses may experience a range of emotion, stress, and even feelings of burnout during this time. Nurse unit leaders are responsible for managing their own emotions, as well as managing the rest of unit nurses. How might mindfulness benefit nurse-unit leaders in reducing some of the negative emotion, stress, or burnout they experience during a long work shift, in addition to the responsibility to manage other nurses?

With a better understanding of employees, mindful leaders are better able to show genuine care and respect to their employees [24]. Previous work suggests that when leaders are more mindful, they are more likely to have a heightened sense of awareness, understanding, and are able to respond mindfully when engaging with their followers [25]. Moreover, followers are more satisfied with mindful leaders due to the improved quality of communication that mindful leaders exhibit [26]. Finally, mindfulness is linked with leaders' ability to adapt to change by better embracing changing situations and focusing on solutions [19]. Considering the benefits of leader mindfulness, it is important for us to explore the ways mindfulness affects leaders of healthcare teams.

9.1.4   Mindfulness at the Team Level

Mindfulness research at the team level has been slower to develop, but recent work has suggested that team mindfulness is the team's belief that team interactions and experiences are mindful [27]. Preliminary research demonstrates that more mindful teams experience less interpersonal conflict and that individual team members are less likely to engage in negative, interpersonal behaviors such as targeted hostility or aggression toward another member [27]. Additionally, we see that team mindfulness strengthens the positive relationship between individual mindfulness and work engagement [28]. In the healthcare space, patient and staff satisfaction improved after healthcare teams received a mindfulness mentoring intervention [29]. This is an interesting start to understanding how mindfulness can influence healthcare teams, but we still have a lot of work to do in this space.

While team level mindfulness research has gotten off to a slower start than individual-level mindfulness, one compelling future direction for work in this area is to focus on the effects of specific mindfulness practices for healthcare team effectiveness. There are two broad categories of mindfulness practices—formal and informal [30]. Formal mindfulness includes scheduling time for a meditation (e.g., body scan, seated meditation, yoga as mindful movement) or participating in a structured mindfulness-based intervention like this Mindfulness for Interdisciplinary Healthcare Professionals (MIHP) course, mindfulness-based stress reduction (MBSR), or mindfulness-based cognitive therapy (MBCT). On the other hand, informal mindfulness entails intentionally engaging in everyday activities with a heightened sense of presence and attention, like washing the dishes, eating, or listening to a colleague. Based on this research, we suggest that mindfulness practices—both formal and informal—will impact how individual team members show up for their teammates and their shared work.

9.2   Cultivating a Mindfulness Practice: Walking Meditation

Sometimes the smallest step in the right direction ends up being the biggest step of your life. Tip toe if you must, but take the step. – Naeem Callaway

9.2.1   Introduction

Walking meditation is a form of mindful movement. For many, sitting completely still and focusing on the mind while feeling emotions such as anger, sadness, or joy could be overwhelming. Instead, engaging in meditation while physically moving at the same time may feel more manageable. The idea in a walking meditation is to try to calm the mind by focusing on the activity of walking itself [5]. Walking meditations can be done indoors or outdoors at your own pace, just make sure you have ample room to move around. Below we offer an adapted 15-minute walking meditation sample script [31]. Note: this walking meditation is the mindful movement practice for this module; as such, there is no yoga-based mindful movement sequence for this module in Chap. 13, as is typically found for the other modules.

9.2.2 Script

For this meditation, find a space quiet outdoors or a space indoors where there is space to walk in small circles.

Turn your attention inwards toward your physical body. First, take a look down at your feet. Separate them about hip-width distance apart. Engage your legs. Hug your core toward your spine. Lift your chest. Notice if your shoulders are creeping up toward your ears. Use your next exhale to relax your shoulders down, and hug your shoulder blades close toward the spine. Gently wiggle your arms and fingers.

Notice the connection your feet make with the ground. Press your feet down and lift up through your head. Stand up a bit taller. Gently close your eyes if you'd like. Take a deep breath in. Exhale out.

Take 3–5 more deep and controlled cycles of breath. Notice any change in your body with each inhale and exhale.

Notice any noises you may hear. Dogs barking, car engines, or the sound of the wind. Notice if you feel any emotion toward these noises. Take one more full cycle of breath.

If your eyes are closed, blink them open. Press down through the balls of your feet, and wiggle your toes. Gently relax your toes down.

Take inventory of your body here. Notice how it feels. Maybe it feels stiff, strong, or heavy.

Start to shift the weight back and forth from your heels to the toes. Move slowly. Now shift side to side.

Gently come back to center. Notice the connection your feet make with the ground. Notice how the earth supports you.

When you are ready, begin slowly walking forward. Your steps can be as small or as big as you want it to be. You can walk as fast or as slow as you want. Whatever you choose, step with intention.

(Allow participants to walk silently for about 3 min)

Pay close attention to your steps. Land your foot gently with each step. Notice how each foot lifts and lowers through space. Notice the weight shift forward from the heels to the toes.

Continue walking, taking deep inhales and exhales, paying close attention to the sound of your breath and the intentional movement of your body.

(Let participants walk silently for about 3 min)

Notice if your mind has started to wander. Are outside thoughts flowing in and out? Take a moment to bring your attention back to the sensations of your steps. As you move through space, focus your attention on each purposeful step forward.

Notice when you are in contact with the earth. And when you are not.

(Let participants walk silently for 1 more minute)

Slowly, find your tall, standing stance. Stand with purpose. Bring your attention back to your breath. Inhale deeply and exhale slowly.

(pause 3–5 breaths)

Once again, take inventory of your physical body. Notice any difference you may feel now. Maybe a bit looser, maybe stronger, or maybe more relaxed.

Allow yourself to feel held by the earth. Take a few more controlled cycles of breath.

Gently start to bring movement back into your body. When you're ready, open your eyes.

9.3   Tips for Sustaining your Mindfulness Practice

As we discussed in Chap. 7/ Module 3, setting goals and creating routines can be essential for enhancing mindfulness in one's personal and professional life. Here, we offer tips for mindful leaders to share with their teams to encourage and support each other in their mindful practices.

1. *Set a goal* (e.g., one walking meditation practice per week) and track your progress. Some days, you can do a full 15-minute practice and other days, you can do a shorter or longer practice. Even just a few minutes is great. It is normal to feel more or less challenged in settling your mind and focusing your attention on some days than other days. That is why we practice!
2. *Find a meditation buddy.* Having a meditation partner can be helpful for two reasons. First, having a buddy will encourage both of you to hold each other accountable. It is easy to get caught up in the "to-do" list and forgo a walking meditation practice. However, if you and your partner schedule time together, you may have more success in following through your commitment to a meditation practice. You and your meditation buddy can meet as frequently as your schedules allow – we suggest meeting at least once a week to develop a sustainable practice. Second, you and your meditation partner will each have different experiences (and indeed no mindful practice is ever the same!), so this provides an opportunity to reflect on your practice and share your experiences with one another. It is not uncommon for meditation to bring about an emotional experience. It can be helpful to process your experience by talking through the emotions that may arise. Some questions to discuss after your meditation include: How did you feel during the meditation? How do you feel now? What differences do you notice from how you felt before your meditation?
3. *Think of your personal goals.* A walking meditation can improve your emotional health and physical health. Taking breaks throughout the day to stand up, walk, or stretch can reduce low back pain and refresh blood flow into the body, while also settling and refocusing the mind.
4. *Experiment!* Try out the different types of mindfulness practice see what works best for you. For example, try both informal (i.e., eating with a heightened sense of awareness) and formal ways (i.e., body scan, seated meditations). If you feel pressed for time, try integrating informal mindfulness practices during your everyday activities as a way of infusing mindfulness into your daily work and living. On the other hand, if you are looking for a bit more guidance on a given day, try a formal mindfulness practice. The following section has some further resources that offer guided meditations.

9.4   Additional Resources

1. *Reading.* Check out books by Jon Kabat-Zinn and other respected authors in the mindfulness sphere (e.g., Sharon Salzberg, Thich Nhat Hanh, Ellen Langer, Dan Harris, Daniel Siegel, and many others). For example, the book by Kabat-Zinn "Wherever You Go, There You Are" explains what mindfulness entails and offers a number of practical suggestions and practices for individuals who are looking to start a mindfulness practice.
2. *Mobile applications.* Several mobile applications (e.g., Calm, Insight Timer, among others) offer free, live meditation sessions and recordings you can do on your own time, as well as a record of your practices in order to track your meditation progress [32, 33]. Many of them offers targeted meditations (i.e., anxiety, stress, improving sleep, mindfulness for parents, etc.), yoga routines, courses, meditation groups, and talks. You can use these apps by yourself, or your team can utilize these apps together and form a meditation group. In addition, activity trackers (e.g., *Fitbit*) may offer meditations and tools to automatically track your progress [34].
3. *Time for team reflection.* Build in time for your team to reflect on various experiences throughout the day at your next team meeting (i.e., after a shift, a project, or after a given period of time (day, week, month). Team members can individually reflect for a few moments, then share their thoughts, feelings, or experiences with a partner or with the larger group. Questions your team could discuss during a debrief include: What went well during the process? What did not go well? Did the team support each other? What could be improved next time?
4. *Mindful moment during safety huddles.* Safety huddles are informal, short meetings that typically take place at the start or end of a healthcare worker's shift [35]. A moment of mindfulness can be implemented during a safety huddle in order for healthcare members to acknowledge their feelings, breath, and what's going on in their minds and bodies. For example, the shift leader can lead a minute of team meditation to encourage team members to reset and refocus.
5. *The Medical Pause by Jonathon Bartels.* This moment of silence is implemented following the death of a patient to honor the moment and offer closure. This can be a mindful response to the stress accompanied from this experience for medical teams. For more details, see: thepause.me.

9.5   Tips for Instructors

To lead others in mindfulness practices, instructors should remember that you too are, and always will be, practicing. There is no end goal of a mindfulness practice, and you do not have to have a perfect mindfulness practice in order to teach others. Rather, teaching and practicing mindfulness are two sides of the same coin.

9.5.1 Mindfulness Meditation

9.5.1.1 Directions for Meditation Leader

As you deliver this meditation, remember to give your students adequate time to breathe in and breathe out. It is natural for us to get caught up in reading the script such that we can forget about the time it takes to actually breathe. Please note that the comments in the brackets (<< >>) are instructions for you. The text is not actually to be read aloud.

This meditation is focused on bringing attention to the nature of your mind and breath.

To get started, find a comfortable seat. If you have a something to assist you such as a supportive cushion, pillow, or yoga block, place it underneath your seat to take some pressure off your legs and low back. Sit with your legs crossed-legged out in front of you, or sit with your heels underneath your hips.

Start to shift your attention inward, toward your body. Notice the connection your legs are making with the earth. Press down through your seat. Place your palms on your lap. For a grounding experience, place them face down. For a receiving experience, place them face up. Hug your belly close to the spine and left your chest.

Let your shoulders roll up then relax them back down toward your spine. Lift your head. Let your eyelids get heavy and focus your gaze on one point in front of you. Or, you may close your eyes fully if you wish. Exhale your breath.

<<Long pause>>

Now bring your attention toward your breath. We will start to breathe with intention. Through your nose, inhale. Let your chest rise and fill up your lungs. Open your mouth, exhale.

Inhale count down from 4—3—2—1. Pause for a moment. Then, through your mouth, exhale your breath as if you were trying to fog up a mirror.

Inhale/Exhale x3.

<<Long pause>>

Continue moving your breath in and out intentionally.

Notice any thoughts that may be running through your mind. Allow them to come to a pause, knowing that they will return later.

For our meditation practice today, please bring into your mind a mantra. A mantra is a short phrase. Keep it simple. This can be something you'd like to manifest in your life, or something you'd like to let go of. For example, a mantra could be "I believe in myself" or "I am strong" or "I want to let go of negative thoughts". Your mind will always believe what you tell it.

<<Long pause>>

We will silently commit to our mantras now with a cycle of breath. Inhale and exhale.

Now that you have your mantra, silently, continue repeating it in your mind. As you inhale, say the first half of your mantra. As you exhale, say the second half of your mantra.

<<Long pause>>

For a moment, bring your attention back toward your body. Sit up a little taller.

Use this moment as an opportunity to return back to your mantra, once again releasing any thoughts that may have come into your mind.

<<Long pause>>

Collectively, we will take a deep breath in, and a slow breath out. Purposefully, repeat your mantra to yourself one last time.

As you move through the rest of your day, keep this mantra close to you. Your mind will always believe what you tell it.

We will close our meditation practice now.

References

1. Mathieu J, Maynard MT, Rapp T, Gilson L. Team effectiveness 1997-2007: a review of recent advancements and a glimpse into the future. J Manag. 2008;34(3):410–76.
2. Burke CS, Stagl KC, Klein C, Goodwin GF, Salas E, Halpin SM. What type of leadership behaviors are functional in teams? A meta-analysis. Leadership Quarterly. 2006;17(3):288–307.
3. Guzzo RA, Dickson MW. Teams in organizations: recent research on performance and effectiveness. Annu Rev Psychol. 1996;47(1):307–38.
4. Kozlowski SW, Ilgen DR. Enhancing the effectiveness of work groups and teams. Psychol Sci Public Interest. 2006;7(3):77–124.
5. Kabat-Zinn J. Wherever you go, there you are: mindfulness meditation in everyday life. Paris: Hachette Books; 2009.
6. Brown KW, Ryan RM. The benefits of being present: mindfulness and its role in psychological Well-being. J Pers Soc Psychol. 2003;84(4):822.
7. Reina CS, Kudesia RS. Wherever you go, there you become: how mindfulness arises in everyday situations. Organ Behav Hum Decis Process. 2020;159:78–96.
8. Dreyfus G. Is mindfulness present-centred and non-judgmental? A discussion of the cognitive dimensions of mindfulness. Contemporary Buddhism. 2011;12(1):41–54.
9. Good DJ, Lyddy CJ, Glomb TM, Bono JE, Brown KW, Duffy MK, et al. Contemplating mindfulness at work: an integrative review. J Manag. 2016;42(1):114–42.
10. Sutcliffe KM, Vogus TJ, Dane E. Mindfulness in organizations: a cross-level review. Annu Rev Organ Psych Organ Behav. 2016;3:55–81.
11. Glomb TM, Duffy MK, Bono JE, Yang T. Mindfulness at work. In: Research in personnel and human resources management. Bingley: Emerald Group Publishing Limited; 2011.
12. Quaglia JT, Braun SE, Freeman SP, McDaniel MA, Brown KW. Meta-analytic evidence for effects of mindfulness training on dimensions of self-reported dispositional mindfulness. Psychol Assess. 2016;28(7):803.
13. Roche M, Haar JM, Luthans F. The role of mindfulness and psychological capital on the Wellbeing of leaders. J Occup Health Psychol. 2014;19(4):476.
14. Grover SL, Teo ST, Pick D, Roche M. Mindfulness as a personal resource to reduce work stress in the job demands-resources model. Stress Health. 2017;33(4):426–36.
15. Hülsheger UR, Alberts HJEM, Feinholdt A, Lang JWB. Benefits of mindfulness at work: the role of mindfulness in emotion regulation, emotional exhaustion, and job satisfaction. J Appl Psychol. 2013;98(2):310–25.
16. Dust SB, Liu H, Wang S, Reina C. The effect of mindfulness and job demands on motivation and performance trajectories across the workweek: an entrainment theory perspective. J Appl Psychol. 2021. In Press. https://doi.org/10.1037/apl0000887
17. Pipe TB, Bortz JJ, Dueck A, Pendergast D, Buchda V, Summers J. Nurse leader mindfulness meditation program for stress management: a randomized controlled trial. JONA J Nurs Adm. 2009;39(3):130–7.

18. Brendel W, Hankerson S, Byun S, Cunningham B. Cultivating leadership dharma: measuring the impact of regular mindfulness practice on creativity, resilience, tolerance for ambiguity, anxiety and stress. J Manag Dev. 2016;35:1056–78.
19. Rupprecht S, Falke P, Kohls N, Tamdjidi C, Wittmann M, Kersemaekers W. Mindful leader development: how leaders experience the effects of mindfulness training on leader capabilities. Front Psychol. 2019;10:1081.
20. Reb J, Chaturvedi S, Narayanan J, Kudesia RS. Leader mindfulness and employee performance: a sequential mediation model of LMX quality, interpersonal justice, and employee stress. J Bus Ethics. 2019;160(3):745–63.
21. Reb J, Narayanan J, Chaturvedi S. Leading mindfully: two studies on the influence of supervisor trait mindfulness on employee well-being and performance. Mindfulness. 2014;5(1):36–45.
22. Pinck AS, Sonnentag S. Leader mindfulness and employee well-being: the mediating role of transformational leadership. Mindfulness. 2018;9(3):884–96.
23. Schuh SC, Zheng MX, Xin KR, Fernandez JA. The interpersonal benefits of leader mindfulness: a serial mediation model linking leader mindfulness, leader procedural justice enactment, and employee exhaustion and performance. J Bus Ethics. 2019;156(4):1007–25. *10.1037/apl0000887*. 18: it is
24. Reb J, Sim S, Chintakananda K, Bhave DP. Leading with mindfulness: exploring the relation of mindfulness with leadership behaviors, styles, and development. In: Mindfulness in organizations: foundations, research, and applications. Cambridge: Cambridge University Press; 2015. p. 256–84.
25. Reina CS. Adapting leader behaviors to achieve follower effectiveness: a mindful approach to situational leadership. Arizona State University; 2015.
26. Arendt JF, Pircher Verdorfer A, Kugler KG. Mindfulness and leadership: communication as a behavioral correlate of leader mindfulness and its effect on follower satisfaction. Front Psychol. 2019;10:667.
27. Yu L, Zellmer-Bruhn M. Introducing team mindfulness and considering its safeguard role against conflict transformation and social undermining. Acad Manag J. 2018;61(1):324–47.
28. Liu S, Xin H, Shen L, He J, Liu J. The influence of individual and team mindfulness on work engagement. Front Psychol. 2020;10:2928.
29. Singh NN, Singh SD, Sabaawi M, Myers RE, Wahler RG. Enhancing treatment team process through mindfulness-based mentoring in an inpatient psychiatric hospital. Behav Modif. 2006;30(4):423–41.
30. Birtwell K, Williams K, van Marwijk H, Armitage CJ, Sheffield D. An exploration of formal and informal mindfulness practice and associations with wellbeing. Mindfulness. 2019;10(1):89–99.
31. Walking Meditation Guided Script [Available from: https://mindfulnessexercises.com/walking-meditation-guided-script/.
32. Calm. Available from: https://www.calm.com/.
33. Insight Timer. Available from: https://insighttimer.com/.
34. Fitbit. Available from: https://www.fitbit.com/global/us/home.
35. Chapman KB. Improving communication among nurses, patients, and physicians. AJN Am J Nurs. 2009;109(11):21–5.

Module 6: Mindful Compassion in the Presence of Suffering

10

Jordan Quaglia

Unlike *mindfulness*, the word *compassion* has long been part of the Western vocabulary, so many people tend to assume they know what it means. However, as we will explore in this chapter—both conceptually and experientially—many of us have grown familiar with ideas and representations of compassion that aren't always consistent with scientific understanding. In other words, we might think we know what compassion looks and feels like, when what we're actually experiencing is something other than compassion per se. This raises a number of interesting questions worth contemplating at the outset of our exploration of compassion, such as: Where do our ideas about compassion from? How do they intersect with, and influence, our day-to-day engagement with being a compassionate person? Do we believe compassion is supportive of our work or do we think compassion's downsides outweigh its benefits?

Given the possibility for preexisting views on compassion, it can be helpful to first spend some time exploring what thoughts, feelings, images, and so on come to mind when we heard the word *compassion*. This will allow us to better compare and contrast any notions we have with the actual science and practice of compassion as presented here. Additionally, this will help us consciously identify and work with possible resistance that may arise as we explore activities and practices for cultivating more compassion.

J. Quaglia (✉)
Naropa University, Boulder, CO, USA
e-mail: jquaglia@naropa.edu

Group Reflection

Breaking into triads or small groups, offer some time for deliberate exploration of any preexisting ideas about compassion.

Reflection #1: When you hear the word, *compassion*, what feelings does it give rise to within your body? Are these feelings more pleasant or unpleasant, heavy or light, warm or cool?

Reflection #2: Think for a moment about some images that come to mind when you reflect on compassion. What are these images and why do you think they are part of your associations with compassion?

Reflection #3: What, in your mind, is a real-world example of compassionate action? What, specifically, makes you believe this is an example of compassion per se?

10.1 Key Concepts

Now that we've explored some of our preexisting views on compassion, let's see how they compare with scientific understanding of some key concepts. Often, confusion about compassion comes from its kinship with other, related terms—especially empathy. Therefore, it's important we not only define compassion from a scientific perspective, but also empathy. Establishing a more precise conceptual understanding of compassion will offer a supportive foundation for more precisely cultivating and experiencing compassion.

10.1.1 Empathy

Empathy is a term that's used to describe a variety of related experiences, such as feeling what others are feeling or thinking ourselves into another's shoes. However, the most common meaning of empathy has to do with people's tendency to share in the internal states of others—what has been called *experience sharing* [1]. This refers to the relatively automatic, effortless capacity of the human nervous system to take in cues from the bodies and facial expressions of others, and thereby come to experience something similar in ourselves. For example, how many can relate to the experience of interacting with someone who's sad, and subsequently finding ourselves sadder as a result? If we're not paying close attention, we might even leave the interaction wondering why we're suddenly feeling sad ourselves, not realizing that we "caught" the sadness of another. Note how this kind of experience sharing doesn't really involve us *deciding* to empathize with others. Rather, empathy seems to happen to us. At times, even without our awareness. This is a large part of what is meant by empathy – as experience sharing – being automatic and subconscious. Because of this automaticity, we have limited control over how much we can dial up or down the degree of empathy.

10.1.2 Compassion

Now that we have a basic definition for empathy, we can better understand compassion. Whereas empathy is more about *subconsciously* feeling *with* the feelings of others, compassion is more about *consciously* feeling *for* what others are struggling with [2]. Yet compassion and empathy are not entirely distinct experiences, hence the potential for confusing the two. Specifically, compassion starts with empathy for suffering before growing into a more conscious, regulated experience. On an experiential level, we might first experience the role of empathy as a kind of receiving, or taking in, the experience of suffering. In contrast to empathy alone, however, compassion does not end there. Through compassion, we shift from receiving to offering, generating feelings of care and affection *for* those suffering, as well as an internal readiness to act to alleviate suffering. Putting these pieces together, we can think of compassion as having three main components, namely (1) greater awareness of suffering, (2) feeling *for* the one who is suffering, and (3) an intentional readiness to alleviate suffering if possible [3, 4]. Through compassion practices and training, we work to familiarize ourselves with each of these three components, expanding our capacity to face suffering in more conscious, regulated ways.

10.1.3 Self-Compassion

Self-compassion teaches us that the scope of compassion need not be limited to other people, but can also include ourselves. However, self-compassion is not fundamentally different than compassion for others. It has the same three main components as compassion generally—awareness of suffering, feeling for the one suffering, and readiness to alleviate suffering—but is directed toward one's own suffering. When people are first introduced to compassion, many say it feels harder to generate compassion for themselves than other people, and this may be especially true for healthcare professionals [cf. 5]. Fortunately, training in other-oriented compassion can familiarize us with the experience of compassion in ways that make it easier to practice self-compassion. In turn, growing and deepening our self-compassion can enrich our compassion for others. This potential synergy between both self- and other-oriented compassion means our compassion training will be incomplete if it's not expanding both compassion for both oneself and others. Through training in both, we may even come to experience more holistic forms of compassion that integrate and blend self- and other-oriented compassion [6].

10.1.4 Empathy Fatigue

Knowing the distinction between empathy and compassion, we can better see how and why people often conflate the two. And it turns out researchers are not immune to this sort of misunderstanding. *Compassion fatigue* is a popular phrase in the scientific literature for describing feelings of exhaustion and fatigue that can arise in care providers due to chronic engagement with empathy for the suffering of others [7, 8]. However, it appears more accurate to call this phenomenon *empathic distress fatigue,* or more simply, *empathy fatigue* [9], since the reported symptoms are consistent with the downsides of empathy, and empathy avoidance [9]. Empathy avoidance may play an important role in empathy fatigue, with research showing how people may commonly try to avoid, or decrease empathy, due to perceived costs of empathizing [1]. Since empathy itself is often subconscious and automatic, trying to override or avoid it may contribute more to empathy fatigue than simply allowing the experience of empathy.

10.2   Tips for Instructors

In exploring the distinction between empathy and compassion, it remains important to remind students that feelings of empathy do not go away during compassion. This is because compassion includes, yet goes beyond, empathy. In first learning compassion, there can be a risk of trying to use compassion as another way to avoid empathy. Yet, as noted earlier, empathy for suffering is indeed an important starting point for compassion. In experiencing compassion, our empathy for suffering generally remains. What changes is that our empathy is put into a broader container that helps buffer against its downsides while preserving its upsides. This is also helpful for understanding why compassion not only helps decrease or temper excess empathy for those who report too much empathy, but can also serve to increase healthy empathy for those who may have lower empathy.

10.2.1   Exploring the Downsides of Avoidance

The so-called White Bear Problem refers to the seemingly paradoxical effects of thought suppression [10]. In this activity (script provided below), students try to *not* think about a white bear for a brief but set period of time (30 s to 1 min). While certain avoidance strategies such as distraction may temporarily succeed, most people find it very challenging to avoid thinking about a white bear. What's more, after the set time period, people may note how white bears can flood the mind due to a kind of rebound effect. This activity can therefore help demonstrate why avoidance of suffering or empathy is not an effective solution, and may even lead to experiencing more of what's avoided. In the context of empathy versus compassion, this demonstrates why turning toward (approach rather than avoidance) is likely to be a more effective strategy when faced with suffering.

Practice for Exploring Downsides of Avoidance Let's all try out a brief activity together, the origin of which we can trace all the way back to the writings of Dostoevsky, in 1863. The basic idea is to give us a bit more insight into the workings of our own minds, and its sometimes paradoxical nature. You might even say this activity will reveal to us when and how we can come to be our own worst enemy.

Close your eyes and, for the next [30 s to 1 min], go ahead and try to *not* think of a white bear.

[Pause for 30 s to 1 min]

Okay, great. Not so easy, right? Some of us may have succeeded, using one strategy or another, to keep the white bear at bay. Most people, however, struggle to *not* think of a white bear for long. What's more, now that we've stopped effortfully trying, notice if the white bear is coming to mind with an even greater frequency.

What did you notice during this activity?

[Pause for sharing]

This is what's called the White Bear Problem in psychology, which refers to the seemingly paradoxical effects of suppression and experiential avoidance [10]. In other words, when we try to avoid an internal experience, we often end up experiencing that thing even more strongly—whether in the moment of trying to avoid the experience, and sometime later, due to a kind of rebound effect after the fact.

Group activity: From empathy avoidance to empathy embrace

We are now going to explore how we experience avoidance versus acceptance in social interactions. Break into dyads, where one person is the "listener" and the other is the "speaker". The speaker should share a *mildly* distressing event in their current lives. Choosing a mildly, rather than intensely, distressing event is key to this activity not creating undue distress. The listener tries to listen *without* offering any supportive social cues such as head nodding, facial expressions, or verbal responses. After each partner takes a turn as the listener without providing supportive social cues, repeat the activity while allowing more natural social cues to be expressed as usual. Discuss the felt difference between suppressing these cues versus expressing them. Which was more effortful? Did you succeed in not expressing supportive social cues, or did some slip through anyways? What can this teach us about our innate empathy, and how exhausting it can be to try and avoid it? [Note to instructors: this is a similar group activity to one practiced in a previous module; in this repeat practice, remind practitioners that the focus today is on the felt-experience of avoidance/ suppression vs the full expression of compassion toward another's experience]

10.3   Mindful Movement

A recommended yoga sequence to complement this chapter's theme is provided in Chap. 13.

10.4   Formal Mindfulness Practice

10.4.1 Transforming Empathy into Compassion

In this practice, we will explore what it feels like to transform empathy for suffering into compassion. Each step of the practice is intended to cultivate the three elements of compassion mentioned earlier, namely (1) awareness of suffering; (2) feeling for the one who is suffering; and (3) an intentional readiness to alleviate suffering, which will take the form of an inner wish during this practice. Although we will take each of these steps in turn, the ultimate goal is to experience them together, as one integrated feeling.

Preparing for Practice The timing of this practice is intended to be flexible, with each step taking anywhere from 1 to 5 minutes, depending on how much time you have. To prepare, it is helpful to remove distractions such as your phone and computer, and to settle into a comfortable posture. Generally, it is best to sit upright if you can, but please do what feels best for you. Lastly, it is up to you whether you choose to do this practice with eyes closed or open. If you choose to keep your eyes open, try relaxing your eyes with a soft gaze.

As part of this practice, you will be asked to bring to mind something that invokes a sense of inner warmth and natural affection. So let's start by taking a moment to explore within our experience and identify something. For example, people find calling to mind a pet or animal can have this effect. If you do not have a pet, but you want to explore this, you can simply try reflecting on the last puppy or kitten you saw. Alternatively, you can think about a child, friend, loved one, a place in nature, the sounds of laughter, or anything else that might bring about this natural warmth and affection within.

Once you have identified something, go ahead and let it go for now as we begin the practice.

Step 1: Awareness of Suffering For the first step in this practice, let's grow in our awareness of some kind of suffering we have recently encountered, seen, or heard about in the news. There's no need to choose something big here, and in fact it's important to start with something smaller that does not overwhelm you with feelings. Nonetheless, the invitation here is to grow in our awareness of something that brings with it a natural sense of empathy for the suffering of one or more people.

Allow yourself to feel what you are feeling, and mindfully notice what it is like to empathize with suffering. You might ask yourself: How is this showing up in my body? What images or thoughts are coming to mind? Has my breathing shifted since bringing this to mind?

Step 2: Feeling for the One Suffering Next, let's return to the image or thought you were asked to call to mind earlier—something that helps you connect with a sense of inner warmth, affection, and care. See if you can hold this in your aware-ness, breathing in and allow this warmth to grow. Take a few moments to rest with these natural feelings.

Resting in this place of inner warmth, bring your awareness back to the suffering you were feeling empathy with earlier. Notice if you can hold this suffering person or persons within the container of this warmth and affection you have cultivated. Each time you exhale, imagine this inner warmth and care flowing out and provid-ing some relief to those you are thinking about.

Step 3: Wishing for Alleviation from Suffering Lastly, let's join this sense of warmth with an inner wish, which we can repeat silently. Here are a few possible phrases, "May you be free from this suffering," "May you experience some relief from this suffering," "May you be well." As you wish, note that you need not iden-tify a way to reduce suffering. *This is not about problem solving or fixing.* Instead, you are simply cultivating this wish as a kind of openness to the possibility of some kind of relief, however, big or small.

If you lose touch with your inner warmth, feel free to return to Step Two at any time, again calling to mind the pet, person, or thing that helps you reconnect with affection and care. Once you have reestablished this sense of warmth, you can con-tinue to repeat an inner wish or wishes to yourself for the next few minutes. May you be free from this suffering," "May you experience some relief from this suffer-ing," "May you be well."

References

1. Zaki J. Empathy: a motivated account. Psychol Bull. 2014 Nov;140(6):1608.
2. Singer T, Klimecki OM. Empathy and compassion. Curr Biol. 2014;24(18):R875–8.
3. Gilbert P. The evolution and social dynamics of compassion. Soc Personal Psychol Compass. 2015;9(6):239–54.
4. Jazaieri H, Jinpa GT, McGonigal K, Rosenberg EL, Finkelstein J, Simon-Thomas E, et al. Enhancing compassion: A randomized controlled trial of a compassion cultivation training program. J Happiness Stud [Internet]. 2013;14(4):1113–26.
5. Neff KD, Knox MC, Long P, Gregory K. Caring for others without losing yourself: an adap-tation of the mindful self-compassion program for healthcare communities. J Clin Psychol. 2020;76(9):1543–62.
6. Quaglia JT, Soisson A, Simmer-Brown J. Compassion for self versus other: a critical review of compassion training research. J Posit Psychol [Internet]. 2020;00(00):1–16.
7. Cavanagh N, Cockett G, Heinrich C, Doig L, Fiest K, Guichon JR, Page S, Mitchell I, Doig CJ. Compassion fatigue in healthcare providers: a systematic review and meta-analysis. Nurs Ethics. 2020;27(3):639–65.
8. Figley CR. Treating compassion fatigue. Treating Compassion Fatigue: Routledge; 2013.
9. Klimecki O, Singer T. Empathic distress fatigue rather than compassion fatigue? Integrating findings from empathy research in psychology and social neuroscience. Pathological altruism. 2012;5:368–83.
10. Wegner DM. Setting free the bears: escape from thought suppression. Am Psychol. 2011;66(8):671.

Module 7: Mindful Compassion in the Face of Imperfection

11

Sarah Ellen Braun and Patricia Anne Kinser

11.1 Key Concepts

11.1.1 Discuss Home Practice

Begin a dialogue about whether participants are having difficulty with maintaining a regular mindfulness practice. If so, discuss challenges with them and give space for other participants to chime in with solutions before offering them up as the instructor. If participants have questions about the practices or development of regular practice, facilitate discussion about the questions that arise, allowing other members of the group to respond before offering guidance as the instructor. For example, if it has not been discussed already, consider asking participants how they talk to themselves during meditation. This conversation will often take on a life of its own, as this is a rich aspect of developing the practice. If applicable, consider sharing your own challenges along these lines and what you have learned, always after allowing other group members to contribute first. Depending on the group dynamics present during this week's session, this may be a good time to discuss maintaining or increasing practice when the group classes come to end (after next session). This will be discussed in the following chapter, but initiating the discussion now may be worthwhile—and probably on their minds already!

S. E. Braun (✉)
Department of Neurology, School of Medicine, Virginia Commonwealth University, Richmond, VA, USA
e-mail: sarah.braun@vcuhealth.org

P. A. Kinser
School of Nursing, Virginia Commonwealth University, Richmond, VA, USA
e-mail: kinserpa@vcu.edu

Group Discussion—Common Workplace Errors and Using Mindfulness Strategies to Improve Performance
Discuss the common mistakes made at work and how mindfulness qualities from Module 1 (see below) can be applied to address them.

- What are common mistakes that are made in medical care? What are often the causes of these mistakes? What are the consequences? How can the qualities of mindfulness be applied to our work to mitigate these errors and to reduce the consequences of guilt, shame, and blame?

Let's review the qualities (values) of mindfulness:

1. *Beginner's mind*: approaching things as new and fresh, as if for the first time, with curiosity—even if they are something we've seen many times before.
2. *Nonjudgment*: impartial observation– not labeling thoughts, feelings, or sensations as good or bad, right or wrong, fair or unfair, but simply taking note of thoughts, feelings, or sensations in each moment.
3. *Nonstriving*: no grasping, aversion to change, or movement away from whatever arises in the moment; not trying to get anywhere other than where you are; don't worry if this one (or any of these concepts) is confusing. And feel free to ask questions! But nonstriving especially can be difficult to understand. Think of a time when you really didn't want to something to happen and it did or a time when you really wanted something and it didn't come to be, these are examples of striving. Practicing nonstriving is a way for us to develop awareness of how our aversions (not wanting something) and desires can create suffering. It doesn't mean we can't want things or that it's bad. It's a reminder to notice.
4. *Letting be*: simply let things be as they are, with no need to try to let go of whatever is present. Or we can keep this simple and say "open" - open to things as they are.
5. *Self-reliance*: see for yourself, from your own experience, what is true or untrue. This is super important. Ask questions. Remember that this is a practice of self-inquiry. You are the only one who can do it for yourself, just as I'm the only one who can do it for myself. We receive guidance from teachers and others, but it's a purely experientially thing. Talking about it won't get us there. We've got to experience for ourselves.
6. *Compassion*: cultivating love for oneself and all beings, with the desire to end suffering and promote happiness for all.

Group Activity: Watch this Ted Talk https://www.youtube.com/watch?v= qmaY9DEzBzI

Discussion Questions on Transparency, Compassion, and Truth in Medical Errors:

- Imagine you are that nurse. What are you feeling?
- What are the necessary resources and qualities to support transparency in the face of medical errors? What kind of protection and support would you need?
- The speaker says she needed an "infusion of truth and compassion" and that the nurses and doctors needed it too. What are your thoughts on this? How can we promote a culture of truth and compassion in our future careers?
- In what domains of life could the principles of transparency, compassion, and learning from mistakes be applied?
- The speaker is advocating for transparency in medicine, which is a system-wide change; what can we do as individuals, as a small group, to encourage this change?

11.1.2 Research on Mindfulness and Patient Safety

Several commentaries have been published proposing theoretical rationale for the potential of mindfulness interventions in HCPs to improve patient safety. However, the empirical evidence remains in its infancy. A review in 2018 from our group found four studies [1], which all reported improvements on patient safety outcomes following a mindfulness intervention in HCPs. Patient safety outcomes included near misses, medication errors, absenteeism, and patient falls. However, these studies were limited methodologically making it difficult to interpret the mindfulness training as the sole mechanism driving these improvements [1]. A more recent study found that trait mindfulness was related to greater triage accuracy among emergency department HCPs [2], however, triage accuracy was assessed using self-report and thus introduces some bias to the findings. Similarly, another recent study found that mindfulness for HCPs was related to improved self-reported patient safety [3]. Taken together these findings provide promise for the effects of mindfulness training on patient safety, purportedly via improved decision-making, reduced clinician bias, and even increased processing speed.

Group Discussion with Panel of Healthcare Professionals

Invite several HCPs who practice mindfulness to serve on this panel discussion (see tips for instructors below). Invite the panelists to discuss the following questions, as well as questions from the participants in the group:

- How do you integrate the principles and practices of mindfulness and compassion into your lives? What are the challenges? What is the benefit to you, personally and professionally?
- What do the following quotes mean to you?

"I have come to believe that caring for myself is a not self-indulgent. Caring for myself is an act of survival." Audre Lorde.
"The road to happiness is paved with self-compassion" Anonymous.

11.1.3 Rededicate to Home Practice

This is an opportunity to remind the group to rededicate themselves to their personal goals of integrating mindful practices into daily life. Reminder to the instructor: we do generally caution against saving the discussion of home practice for the end unless you are very confident in your time management abilities, as it can be very easy for this to get sidelined if left toward the end.

11.2   Mindful Movement Practice

A recommended yoga sequence to complement this chapter's theme is provided in Chapter 13.

11.3   Formal Meditation Practices

11.3.1 Tonglen Meditation

Before leading a tonglen meditation, it is our recommendation that you provide a brief description of the practice and its purpose. This could come from your own experience or you could draw from the description in Sect. 3.6 of Chap. 3.

We will begin by resting our mind on a feeling of openness and space. [*Pause*] You may call to mind a feeling of connection to all those who have practiced meditation and wished for the end of suffering, before you, as well as a feeling of connection with all those around the globe who are practicing right now, with you. All the while resting in a sense of spaciousness and openness to the unlimited compassion of this world. [*Pause*].

Now, allow yourself to breathe in a feeling of heaviness, darkness. Breathe this in with each inhale and breathe out openness, lightness, a feeling of freshness. [*Pause*] Continue in this way for a moment, breathing in a sense of heaviness and darkness, and breathing out, relaxing out, lightness, and openness. Work with these textures and your breathing at your own pace. [*Pause 20 s*].

Now, choose a painful situation in your life that is very real to you. This could be the suffering of a loved one, perhaps someone you love is struggling with a disease or undergoing chemotherapy, perhaps someone you know is suffering from depression or stressful times. This could be any situation of suffering or pain that is on your mind and near to your heart. [*Pause*] If you feel stuck or if your own painful situation comes to mind quickly, work with your own feeling of pain and suffering.

Perhaps you are struggling with jealously or recently lost someone you love. Perhaps you were recently diagnosed with a disease. Whatever painful situation you choose, whether it's someone you know or your own, breathe the pain and suffering in, almost like opening to the pain. You open your breath, heart, and mind to this experience of suffering. This, too, can find a place of belonging in the vast openness of your heart. Now, breathe out relief from that suffering. Breathe out, relax out, healing, and peace. [*Pause*] Breathing in, opening the heart to receive the suffering; breathing out, sending out relief and healing. [*Pause 10 s*].

Begin to grow the target of this sending and receiving. Breathing in this specific type and experience of pain and suffering from a group of others, and breathing out, sending out, relief and healing to an ever-expanding group. [*Pause*] Continue growing the target, eventually receiving this particular pain from everyone who is experiencing it and sending out, relaxing out, relief, and healing to all. [*Pause 15 s*]. You can continue growing out—breathing in, receiving the suffering and breathing out, sending relief to all beings everywhere.

11.3.2 Tips for instructors: Organizing a Panel of Speakers

The aim of this panel is to gather together multiple healthcare professionals from various disciplines who have an active mindfulness and compassion practice integrated into their lives. It is not necessary but it is ideal if they have engaged in a mindfulness curriculum in the past, whether this one or a mindfulness-based stress reduction (MBSR) or similar curriculum. Invite healthcare professionals that you know or reach out to your colleagues for help to identify appropriate individuals. Try to seek out individuals from a variety of disciplines, from nursing to medicine to social work to psychology and beyond. When you invite them to the panel, provide a brief summary of this curriculum on Mindfulness for Interdisciplinary Healthcare Professionals (for example, you might share aspects of Chaps. 1, 2, 3, and 4). Ask them to come to discuss how they have applied mindfulness and compassion practices to the challenges of working in healthcare. Invite them to be honest about their personal process. The panel topics should be broad and largely guided by the participants' questions as well as the experiences of those on the panel.

References

1. Braun SE, Kinser PA, Rybarczyk B. Can mindfulness in health care professionals improve patient care? An integrative review and proposed model. Transl Behav Med. 2019;9(2):187–201. https://doi.org/10.1093/tbm/iby059.
2. Saban M, Dagan E, Drach-Zahavy A. The Relationship Between Mindfulness, Triage Accuracy, and Patient Satisfaction in the Emergency Department: A Moderation-Mediation Model. J Emerg Nurs. 2019;45(6):644–60. https://doi.org/10.1016/j.jen.2019.08.003.
3. Hofert SM, Tackett S, Gould N, Sibinga E. Mindfulness instruction for community-hospital physicians for burnout and patient care: A pilot study. J Patient Safety Risk Manag. 2020;25(1):15–21. https://doi.org/10.1177/2516043519897830.

Module 8: Finding Balance Through Mindful Living

12

Lisa Phipps and Evan Cameron

12.1 Key Concepts

> **Group Discussion: Let's Talk About Home Practice**
> Throughout this mindfulness journey, we have explored several different practices. Let's take a few moments to reflect upon these practices:
>
> - Which resonated well with you? Which ones did not?
> - Which might you continue to do, and which ones will you likely not try again?
> - Are there any that you might modify for yourself?
> - What thoughts and feelings are going into this decision process?
> - Have you considered creating goals for maintaining practice beyond this class? How will you evaluate them in the next few weeks?

12.1.1 What Does Balance Mean?

When we think about the concept of balance, several words or phrases might come to mind: equilibrium, stability, harmony, homeostasis, even distribution, and others. We often talk about being in or out of balance or maintaining balance. Is being "in balance" truly possible? Is it sustainable?

L. Phipps (✉)
Clinical Care Options, Richmond, VA, USA
e-mail: lphipps@clinicaloptions.com

E. Cameron
Richmond Complementary and Integrative Health, Richmond, VA, USA
e-mail: evan.cameron@rcihealth.com

Consider the image of a counterweight scale, and what it means for it to be in balance. In that image, everything must be still, unmoving, seemingly frozen in time. Life, however, is not static. In this way, balance is not the goal, but instead, the teacher. Each day is not the same as the one before-- events come up that change our routines. If we can consider being "in balance" as more of a state in which we must manage the ups and downs and *flow* of life, we can be more forgiving of ourselves and others when things do not go as planned. In this way, we can work toward maintaining balance by managing the sway, the flow of life with a sense of calm and confidence.

Group Activity
Watch this 2.5 min video: "Balance is the wrong analogy"—Simon Sinek, LinkedIn Speaker Series 2019.
   Discuss the following questions:

- What is your response, in general?
- Do you agree with him that "balance" is the wrong analogy, when thinking about work-life balance?
- Is it possible to disconnect completely, as he suggests? Why or why not?
- Which phrase resonates most with you: being "in balance", or being able to "flow" with life?

12.1.2 More on Balance and Flow

Throughout this curriculum, we have explored the concepts of positive stress and negative stress, and signs of burnout. Just as we would want a patient to continue taking their medications even if their blood pressure has improved, we need to remember to maintain our practice even if we are feeling like things are going really well. Have you ever said to yourself—"I'm feeling really good today, so I don't need to meditate"? Pay attention to this tendency to skip your mindful practices. Remember that we practice on the good days and on the tough days. Just as we might lift weights on a regular basis to maintain muscle strength, we must maintain regular practice to maintain the mindful muscle.

Also, regular practice makes it much easier to recognize early signs of burnout or when the shift in stress is starting to affect us. Regular practice allows us insights into what we need at any given time to support ourselves—whether to keep our habits or intensify our practice as we need to. As our lives shift and change, our practice may also look different at times. We may add a practice, or change one that does not seem to be working well for us. It is incredibly important to allow for the recognition that something is changing, without judgment of it, and to consider how to get ourselves back on track. When talking to yourself about it, notice your thoughts and consider whether what you are saying to yourself is something you would say to a friend, family member, or patient.

12.1.3 Getting Ourselves "Unstuck"

It is natural that, during the flow of life, one might feel "stuck" and struggle with maintaining a regular mindfulness practice. One suggestion for getting back on track, or when we are in a place of feeling stuck on an obstacle or challenge, is the practice of mental contrasting with implementation intentions, also known as "WOOP" (Wish, Outcome, Obstacle, Plan). Developed and studied by Oettingen and colleagues, research has shown that this process can be effective for helping to manage stress in healthcare professionals [1]. Available as an app or online at the WOOP website (https://woopmylife.org/), this is a 5–10 min process that walks you through a series of questions asking you to consider something you want to accomplish, how that would feel, what inner obstacles are holding you back, and an if/then plan. The answers to these questions result in a short mantra and reminder. Try it out and see what you think!

As has been discussed in previous modules, gratitude practices can also help with getting "unstuck." Research has shown that these kinds of practices can increase engagement and mindfulness and may help to get us unstuck if we are having trouble managing flow or are shifting too much toward negative stress and thinking [2]. Finding or seeking gratitude in our lives daily can be one way of helping us to refocus on priorities, put things in perspective, and increase our positive energy. Try every day, somewhere at the end of your day, to think back on it and find a moment for which you are thankful. It could be a conversation you had with someone, something in nature that you noticed, or a song that made you smile. The idea is to find the small things, rather than creating a laundry list of the big things, though on some days, these may also provide us with some perspective. If it is helpful, write them down, either in a journal or just as a phrase on a calendar, so that you can look back at them. Also, check out the collection of practices in the Greater Good in Action site (https://ggia.berkeley.edu/). The site suggests first listing five things that make your life happy and enjoyable, to get your mind into a realm of positive thinking. Next, consider a time when something did not go well, and describe that in a few sentences. Finally, list three things that could help you to see the bright side of the situation. Participating in an exercise like this can help us to reevaluate when things do not seem to be going our way or when we are feeling particularly stuck or frustrated.

Another mindful practice that can help one stay connected and mindful of the positive aspects of life is the "Three Good Things" exercise. Research suggests that, when completed daily for at least a week, there are important positive effects in one's life [3]. It's a simple practice: write in detail at the end of each day about three good things that happened that day. The writing should include a brief title or description of what happened, then as much detail about the situation and circumstances around the event, how it made you feel then, how you are feeling about it now as you write about it, and why you think it happened. A team, couple, or family variation on this could include a discussion in which everyone picks one or two good things and talks about them. This can also be combined with gratitude practices, as there is plenty of overlap.

12.1.4 Group Activity: Brief "Finding Balance" Practice

Let's stand up and bring a little blood flow into our legs. Now choose a pose that requires some level of physical balance; popular ones might include the yoga tree or a chi-gong breathing pose, pictured below in Fig. 12.1.

Note that these poses may be difficult for many to hold for much longer than 30 seconds to a minute. The point of this exercise is to recognize changes and shifts in balance, and when we start to feel like we are losing the sense of balance.

Hold the pose and breathe naturally, focusing on taking an inventory of the physical body. What feels balanced, and what changes as you shift your focus and breathing? Are there areas of tension, relaxation, or discomfort? What muscles are engaged and working, and which do not need to be? Does one side of the body feel different from the other? Take note of your heart rate. Now try holding your breath and note what changes (pause for several seconds). Next try focusing on breathing deeply and note what changes (pause for a few breath cycles). Take note of when you feel you are starting to lose your sense of balance. Try putting your foot back down, resetting, and lifting the other foot. How do the feelings of balance change when you switch sides?

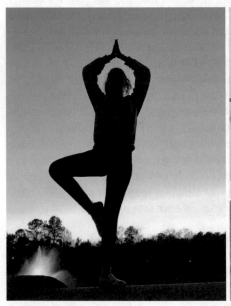 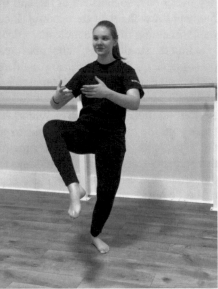

Fig. 12.1 Standing balancing poses. *Picture on Left*: Tree Pose. *Instructions*- Start standing and shift your weight over to one leg. Bend the opposite knee, bringing it out to the side. Bring your foot to either your ankle, calf or thigh, but avoid the knee. This can also be done with the toes resting on the earth and the heel against your opposite ankle, if there is risk of falling. *Picture on Right*: Chi-gong pose. *Instructions*- Stand with feet shoulder's width apart, put one foot forward, lift it, round off arms, bend standing knee slightly. This can also be done with the foot just very lightly touching the ground if there is risk of falling

As you come to a standing pose again, consider how the practice of a balancing pose like this helps to simulate the process of facing challenges in our daily life. In our daily lives, we must notice when we feel a little "wobbly," when we're feeling a bit unbalanced. We must recognize when our ego is getting in the way because we do it to "look good." We must recognize that it is all part of our practice—to recognize, to re-engage, and to move with the flow of life in a healthy way.

> **Group Discussion: Wrapping-Up and Moving Forward—What Will be My Everyday Routine?**
>
> In our opening discussion today, we reflected on the various practices we have explored, which ones worked well for us or did not, and why, and we set some goals for maintaining practice. Next, we experienced some practices that explored the concepts of balance and flow, physically, emotionally, and mentally.
>
> Knowing that "life happens," our routines will be disrupted, and that things will shift and change on us, what are some ways you will note when you need to refocus and re-center, re-instate a practice, or perhaps change or modify one? What resources will you access to help yourself stay committed to your mindful practices?

12.2 Tips for Instructors

Remember that, at this point in the curriculum, the participants should be encouraged to do the majority of the talking/ discussing. Avoid jumping in to give examples during group discussions. Let the participants lead the dialogue. Refocus the conversation if needed, but otherwise be mindful of your need to control the discussion.

12.3 Mindful Movement

A recommended yoga sequence to complement this chapter's theme is provided in Chap. 13.

12.4 Formal Mindfulness Practice

12.4.1 Option 1: Guided Imagery: Exploring Balance and Flow

This visualization exercise is designed to explore the concepts of balance and flow through taking us on a brief journey down a stream. The script below should be read with a calming voice, beginning at a fairly normal pace but slowing, with appropriate pauses during breathing to allow for longer breaths. At the end of the exercise, to help bring people back to external awareness, the last few sentences should be read with slightly increasing speed, energy, and volume, back to normal speaking cadence.

12.4.1.1 Script

Find a comfortable position. Begin by taking deep breaths. Push out your abdomen as you inhale, and pull in your abdomen as you exhale (allow them a few moments to get comfortable with this breathing pattern.) On your next exhale, close your eyes. (pause to allow time to react) As you inhale, open your eyes. Exhale and close your eyes (pause)...inhale and open them. Exhale and close. Inhale and open. Continue this pattern on your own as you continue to breathe deeply. (Pause to allow them to continue for a few moments on their own.) On your next exhale, close your eyes and let them stay closed. Allow your breathing to normalize as you focus your attention on your eyelids. Imagine the energy in your eyelids becoming calm. As your energy stills you feel your eyelids becoming relaxed and heavy. Let the room start to fade away around you with each breath. (pause for a few deep breath cycles). Imagine yourself in your favorite woods. Notice the trees around you, how thick the foliage is above your head, and see the beautiful trees and plants all around you. Take in the rays of light as they make their way through the canopy creating dramatic light and dark patches in the woods around you. Take a deep breath in and exhale. Close your eyes and feel the sunlight and the breeze. Inhale deeply and take in the smell of the forest. Wonderful. And as you open your eyes in the forest, you see in front of you a bright ray of light illuminating a beautiful, still pool of water. As you walk up to the pool, you notice the soft, green moss that is growing right up to its edge, and the beautiful flowers growing all around it. You decide to put your feet in, and as you do. The water feels calm and inviting. Your feet feel almost instantaneously relaxed and comfortable, and that feeling seems to be spreading all over your body. I want you now to imagine yourself gently sliding into this pool and as the water moves up your body, you feel the comforting, inviting feeling of the water as your muscles relax, as your energy becomes still and calm, and as you slide all the way in and allow yourself to float in the water, you feel comfortable. You feel still. You feel your mind, your emotions, all becoming very calm, very relaxed, and very still. You feel your energy settling. You feel your mind becoming very open and clear. You feel your body, your mind, and your spirit resetting. You feel comfortable and relaxed, and you notice that there above you, is a loose branch on a tree. And as the breeze blows, some of the leaves and twigs, and that branch come loose and fall into the pool. And they it hit the water, you feel the ripples gently move across you, but the water has protected you as you float along with its ups and downs. You felt the presence of the branch falling, but you were more than able in this wonderful pool to handle the ripples of water that were created by the impact and you're feeling comfortable, relaxed and at ease. As you find yourself resetting, you find the relaxation rejuvenating, causing you to feel more and more capable of doing the things you want. You look around and notice that this pool has been created by sticks and rocks that have blocked a stream that is gently running into the pool. And now that you are feeling balanced, relaxed, calm, and still, you move your body over to the rocks and sticks that are blocking the path of the stream and you begin to remove them. As you remove them, you feel the water begin to move and flow. You let your body relax and you begin to move and flow with the water. The water hasn't left you. It is still there to protect you, soothe you, relax you, but you are now moving with it. Moving down the stream, feeling comfortable, feeling relaxed, feeling so in control of yourself. The water moves you up and down, left and right, as it follows its path. You notice the movement, enjoying it and being mindful of it. Take a few moments to enjoy this feeling of being in control of yourself while still moving along with the flow of the water. Good. (pause for a minute). You find that as you move along, the water begins to still again, and it is starting to create another pool. And you have had such fun moving up and down in the water as it moved you along, that it feels good now for the pool to stop your motion, as you just lie there, floating in the water, feeling the bright sunlight on your face, as you let the water soothe, relax, and comfort you. You feel good, you feel balanced, you feel in control. You feel yourself coming to a marvelous point where your mind, your body, your emotions, and your spirit, are all relaxed, calm, and balanced. You put your feet down on the bottom of the pool and you stand up and look around. You notice how beautiful the scenery is around you. The gorgeous trees, the beautiful flowers, the wonderful clear color of the water as the light reflects off of it. You notice that this pool too has some sticks and rocks that are slowing the flow of the water down the stream. You know that then you are ready to start your journey again, you have the ability to move those sticks and rocks, to embrace the flow of the water, feeling confident, in control, and in balance as you move with it. You can manage this journey. Take a few moments to enjoy this feeling of confidence and motivation you have created for yourself. (pause few moments). (begin changing voice back to normal speed, volume, and cadence with each sentence). Now I want you to take a deep breath in, and exhale. And another... And on this next deep breath in, start feeling the room coming back around you, as the forest and stream disappear for now, though you know that they are there for you at any time. You feel confident in your abilities to manage your journey, and begin to feel energetic as you take another breath in and open your eyes, feeling relaxed, and good, and ready to move forward in your day.

12.4.2 Option 2: Body Scan Progressive Relaxation

The Body Scan is a progressive relaxation exercise that systematically draws attention to areas of the body to release tension there. This script should be read with a calming voice, beginning at a fairly normal pace but slowing, with appropriate pauses during breathing to allow for longer breaths. At the end of the exercise, to help bring people back to external awareness, the last paragraph should be read with slightly increasing speed, energy, and volume, back to normal speaking cadence. This exercise can also be useful for mindful rest in preparation for sleep, without the return to wakefulness.

12.4.2.1 Script

Find a comfortable position. Begin by taking deep breaths. Push out your abdomen as you inhale, and pull in your abdomen as you exhale. (allow them a few moments to get comfortable with this breathing pattern. Good. On your next exhale, close your eyes. (pause to allow time to react). As you inhale, open your eyes. Exhale and close your eyes (pause)...inhale and open them. Exhale and close. Inhale and open. Continue this pattern on your own as you continue to breathe deeply. (Pause for a full minute) On your next exhale, close your eyes and let them stay closed. Good. Allow your breathing to normalize as you focus your attention on your eyelids. Imagine the energy in your eyelids becoming calm. As your energy stills you feel your eyelids becoming relaxed and heavy.

Move your attention to your forehead, cheeks, and chin. Think about letting go of the tension in your face. Feel your jaw muscles relax allowing the tension to drift away. Feel your cheeks let go of any tension they are carrying as your face begins to feel like it is elongating. Now move your attention down to your neck and shoulders. So many of us carry stress in our neck and shoulders. As you think about the tension in your muscles relaxing you find that any stress you are feeling reduces. Focus your attention on relaxing the muscles in this area. Allow all other thoughts to drift to the back of your mind. Clearing your mind can be hard to do. It is okay if you find that it is. Just focus on the muscles in your neck and shoulders and think about them relaxing. Other thoughts may be present but let them run in the background. Allow yourself this time to focus on resetting your mind, body, and emotions. Move your attention down your arms. As you slowly move your attention think about letting go of the tension in the muscles. Feel your arms getting heavy as your energy becomes still and you feel your relaxation increase. Move your attention down into your wrist, hands, and fingertips. As you think about those muscles relaxing you find that your energy flows out of your fingertips taking with it any tension or stress you have in this area of your body. As you let the energy go you find that you become more relaxed. The comfort and relaxation you are creating for yourself is making the idea of moving hard to entertain. Shift your attention to your back. Starting at the top and working your way down, allow the muscles to let go of tension and stress. Imagine your energy in this area slowing down and becoming very still. As these muscles relax you find that your body feels like it is sinking into whatever you are sitting or lying on. That is okay. Embrace this feeling and allow it to do the job of supporting you so that your muscles do not need to work so hard. Now think about the muscles in your chest and abdomen. As you focus on these muscles relaxing you find that your breath naturally gets deeper. This brings more oxygen into your body, aiding you in the relaxation process. As you give yourself this chance to relax and reset you find that unrelated thoughts are moving further into the background. Your mind is becoming very still. Your body is becoming very relaxed. Your emotions are becoming very balanced. Move your attention to your legs. Imagine those muscles letting go of tension and stress. Feel your energy in your legs becoming very still. We put so much wear and tear on our legs through the course of the day. As you feel these muscles relaxing you find the stress drift away allowing these muscles the chance to recover. You find that as your energy stills in this area of your body, the idea of moving becomes more off-putting. You can move if you need to; however, the idea is becoming more difficult to entertain. Now focus on the muscles in your feet and toes. As these muscles let go of tension and stress, you find a wave of relaxation washes over you. From the top of your head to the tips of your toes, this wave takes with it any remaining tension and stress leaving you feeling completely relaxed and comfortable. You are now feeling in complete control over your mind, body, and emotions. Take a few minutes to enjoy this opportunity and feeling you have created for yourself. (pause for a few minutes). As you embrace the relaxation you have created for yourself, feel your mind, body, and emotions resetting. You are taking a little time to better prepare yourself to mentally, emotionally, and physically handle the tasks you have ahead of you. In just a moment you will begin to shift your attention away from your body. Even after you do you will find that the relaxation you have created for yourself will stay with you. You will continue to feel in control of your mind, body, and emotions. Before you shift your attention take one last moment to embrace the relaxation and comfort you have created from yourself. (increase speed and volume of your voice slightly) Now think about your energy increasing. As you do, you find that your body begins to move. Your thoughts begin to focus on the sound of the room. Your attention is coming back to the things around you. When you are ready go ahead and open your eyes. (Allow a quiet moment for people to open their eyes and adjust to the light. If people are not opening their eyes just repeat the last two lines.)

References

1. Gollwitzer PM, Mayer D, Frick C, Oettingen G. Promoting the Self-Regulation of Stress in Health Care Providers: An Internet-Based Intervention. Front Psychol. 2018;9:838. https://doi.org/10.3389/fpsyg.2018.00838. PMID: 29962979; PMCID: PMC6013563
2. Sergeant S, Mongrain M. An online optimism intervention reduces depression in pessimistic individuals. J Consult Clin Psychol. 2014;82(2):263–74.
3. Seligman ME, Steen TA, Park N, Peterson C. Positive psychology progress: Empirical validation of interventions. Am Psychol. 2005;60(5):410.

Summary of Mindful Movement Sequences

13

John Salisbury, Jennifer Huberty, Mariah Sullivan, Nicole Curtin, and Sarah Ellen Braun

13.1 Introduction to Leading Yoga

It is important to invite a trained yoga instructor (at least 200 h Registered Yoga Teacher (RYT)) to teach the mindful movement portion of this book. They can provide some brief background in regards to the importance of cultivating mindfulness in movement and developing a yoga practice alongside a seated meditation practice. We provide the following sequences, written by an RYT instructor (500+ hours), as potential guides to lead a class in mindful movement aligned with the theme of each curriculum module/chapter. However, if you are working with a trained yoga instructor, we encourage you to allow them to create their own sequences and teach what they know. Please make use of the pictures of the yoga poses as needed.

All yoga poses may be done with ujjayi breathing (see yoga breathing, item 13.2.2 below) and held for approximately 30 s or 10 breaths. Props such as blankets,

Photos used with permission by Nicole Curtin Photography.

J. Salisbury
Modern Yoga, Scottsdale, AZ, USA
e-mail: john@modern.yoga

J. Huberty (✉)
Calm, San Francisco, CA, USA
e-mail: jen@calm.com

M. Sullivan
College of Health Solutions, Arizona State University, Tempe, AZ, USA
e-mail: msulli27@asu.edu

N. Curtin
Nicole Curtin Photography, Phoenix, AZ, USA
e-mail: info@nicolecurtinphotography.com

S. E. Braun
Department of Neurology, School of Medicine, Virginia Commonwealth University, Richmond, VA, USA
e-mail: sarah.braun@vcuhealth.org

pillows, bolsters, and blocks may be used to support individualized practice, particularly for participants who are newer to yoga practice and for those who prefer a gentle/ supported style of practice.

13.2   Chapter 5 Module 1: Intro to Mindfulness

1. **Supta Baddha Konasana**

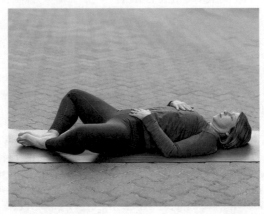

    (a) **Instructions**: Lie on the floor, with the knees bent and open and the bottom of your feet together and hand on chest and belly. [Note: props such as pillows, blankets, bolsters, and/or blocks can be used to support the back and hips, as needed]

    (b) **Benefits**: Grounding, energizing, stress relief, stretches, and opens the hips.

2. **Yoga breathing or ujjayi pranayama (no picture)**

    (a) **Instructions**: Find a comfortable seated position. Close your mouth and slightly constrict the back of the throat, creating an ocean-like sound. Begin with a short exhale, then inhale smoothly with the same constriction in the throat. It will sound like rolling waves of the ocean. Do this 10 times. Continue to breath in the manner during all poses.

    (b) **Benefits**: Improves concentration, builds heat in the body.

3. **Tadasana** (active savasana)
   a. Arms by side

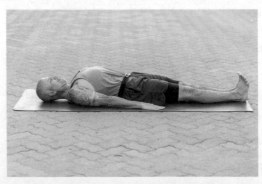

b. Arms over head

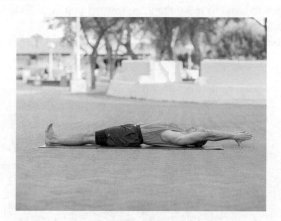

(a) **Instructions**: Lie on your mat with your feet together and actively squeeze your legs. Arms can reach either toward your feet or overhead.
(b) **Benefits**: Grounding pose that energizes the body and opens the chest.

4. **Lying twist**

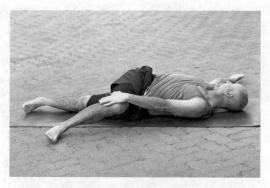

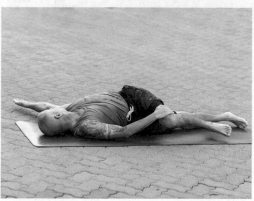

(a) **Instructions:** Lie on your back and bring one knee toward your chest. Use the opposite hand to draw the knee toward that side. Extend the other arm out in a T shape.

(b) **Benefits:** Stretches your back, hips, and glutes, and helps the body to relax.

5. **Cat/Cow**

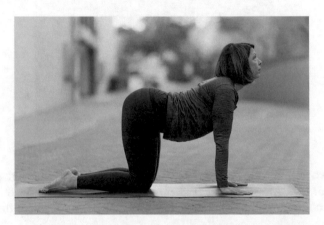

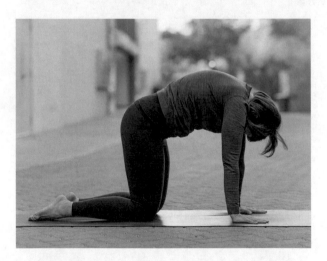

(a) **Instructions:** Start on your hands and knees in a tabletop position. As you inhale, look up, pulling chest forward, flip butt up, and lift your chest. As you exhale, round the back and shoulders as you gaze at navel.

(b) **Benefits:** Strengthens and stretches your spine. Improves focus on body and breath.

6. **Down dog**

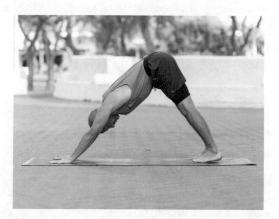

(a) **Instructions:** Start on your hands and knees in a tabletop position. Walk your hands out and lift your hips up and back until you're in an inverted V shape. Keep your back flat – it's ok to bend your knees!
(b) **Benefits:** Stretches the back you're the legs and strengthens the entire body. Good for anxiety relief. Considered a resting pose.

7. **Walk to front of mat – stand**

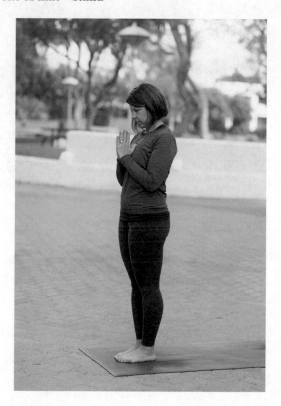

(a) **Instructions:** Stand at the front of your mat with your feet as wide as your hips. Arms can be by your sides or hand together in front of your chest.

(b) **Benefits:** Improves balance and posture. Grounding.

8. **Half vinyasa**

   a. Inhale hands up

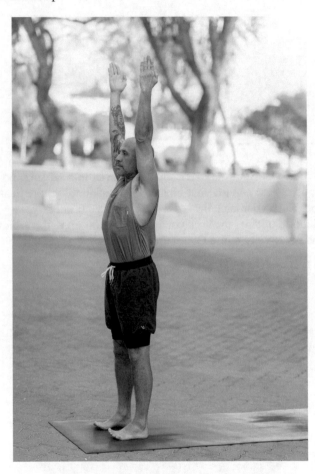

b. Forward fold exhale

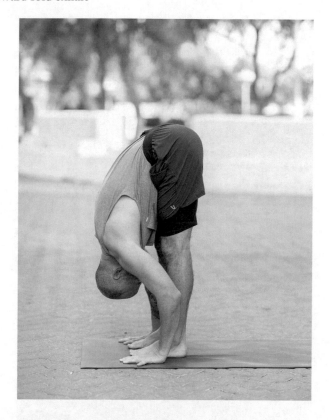

c. Inhale, head up, exhale, forward fold

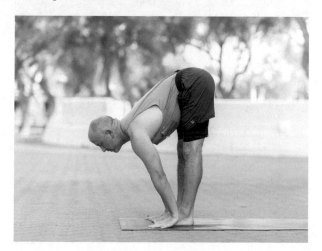

d. Inhale rise back up with arms overhead

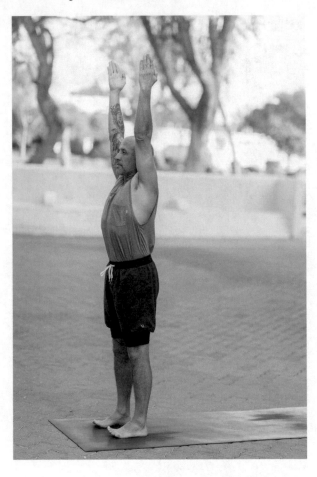

e. Exhale, tadasana standing

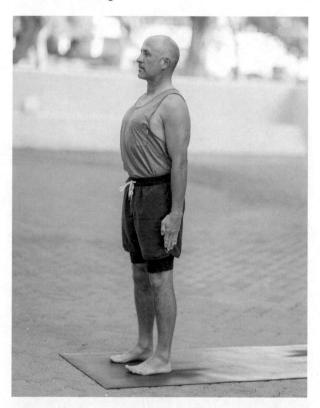

(a) **Instructions**:

   a. As you inhale, lift your arms above your head keeping your ribs neutral (not lifting or splayed).

   b. As you exhale, hinge at the hips as you fold forward. Place hands on ankle or floor, you can bend your knees. If your hands do touch the floor, try to flatten your hand to the floor in the same line as your toes.

   c1. As you inhale, lift your head placing hands on floor or on your shins and extend your spine.

   c2. As you exhale, return to your fold forward. Your hands do not need to touch the floor and you can bend your knees.

   d. As you inhale, return to your first standing position, Lift your arms above your head keeping your ribs neural (not lifting or splayed).

   e. As you exhale, return your arms to your sides.

(b) **Benefits:** Increases blood flow, builds heat, and boosts energy.

9. **Locust pose**

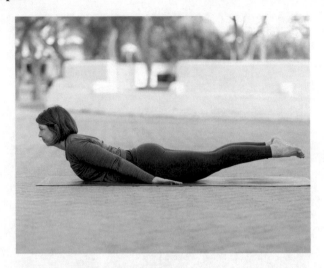

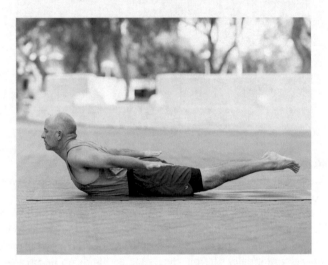

(a) **Instructions:** Start lying face down. Lift your chest, arms, and legs using the strength of your back and glutes.

(b) **Benefits:** Strengthens the back of the body and stretches the front. Helps improve posture and relieve stress.

10. **Tadasana** (active savasana)
    a. Arms by side

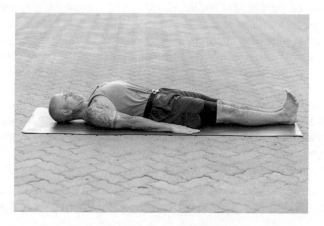

    b. Arms over head

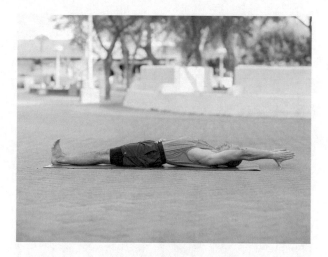

    (a) **Instructions**: Lie on your mat with your feet together and actively squeeze
    your legs. Arms can reach either toward your feet or overhead.

    (b) **Benefits**: Grounding pose that energizes the body and opens the chest.

11. **Savasana**

    (a) **Instructions**: Lie on your back with legs extended (if there is any pain/
    discomfort in the low back, bend the knees, planting the feet on the floor.
    Take the feet a little bit wider than hip distance and allow the knees to fall
    toward each other). Close the eyes. Breathe normally (allow the ujjayi
    breath to fade). Rest the body completely. Allow the mind to rest. As they

come into consciousness, gently let go of thoughts, feelings, and any tension that may arise. (Pause) Practice resting. Letting go. (Pause). First we let go of our physical bodies, relaxing and releasing any tension. (Pause). Then we let go of any tension in our mental and emotional bodies. We practice surrender. (Long pause). Gently begin to wiggle fingers and toes. Perhaps stretching the body as if waking from a deep sleep. Hug the knees into the chest and roll over on one side. Take a moment here. Then press up to come to sitting, opening the eyes slowly.

(b) **Benefits**: Deep rest and relaxation are underemphasized in our world. But rest is an important counterpart to movement. Practicing letting go reduces tension, improves bodily awareness, and provides us with nourishing energy.

13.3   Chapter 6 Module 2: Enhancing Resilience and Burnout

1. **Tadasana standing**

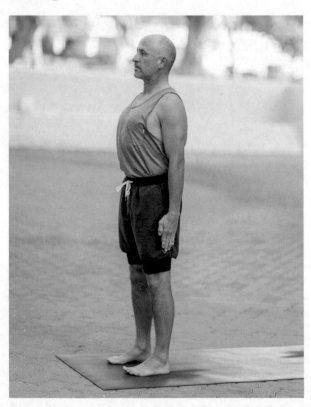

(a) **Instructions:** Stand at the front of your mat with your feet as wide as your hips. Arms can be by your sides or hand together in front of your chest.

(b) **Benefits**: Improves posture and balance.

2. **Half vinyasa**

a. Inhale hands up

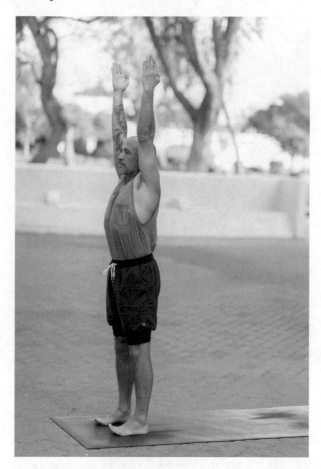

b. Forward fold exhale

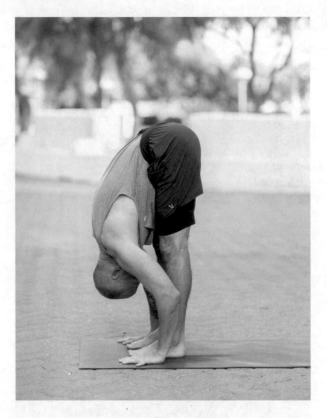

c. Inhale, head up, exhale, forward fold

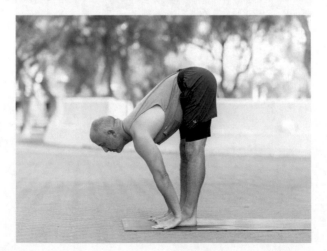

d. Inhale rise back up with arms overhead

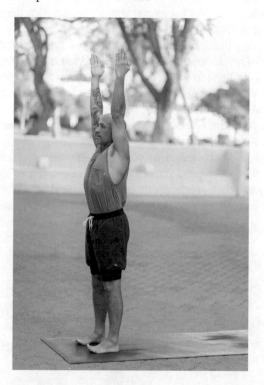

e. Exhale, tadasana standing

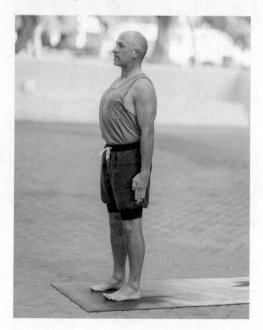

(a) **Instructions:**

   a. As you inhale, lift your arms above your head keeping your ribs neutral (not lifting or splayed).

   b. As you exhale, hinge at the hips as you fold forward. Place hands on ankle or floor, you can bend your knees. If your hands do touch the floor, try to flatten your hand to the floor in the same line as your toes.

   c1. As you inhale, lift your head placing hands on floor or on your shins and extend your spine.

   c2. As you exhale, return to your fold forward. Your hands do not need to touch the floor and you can bend your knees.

   d. As you inhale, return to your first standing position, Lift your arms above your head keeping your ribs neural (not lifting or splayed).

   e. As you exhale, return your arms to your sides.

(b) **Benefits:** Increases blood flow, builds heat, and boosts energy.

3. **Fierce pose** (chair) hands up

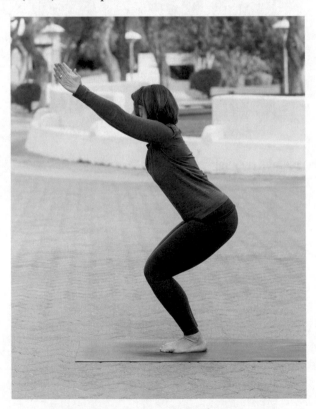

(a) **Instructions:** Bring your knees and feet together. Bend your knees and sink your hips back, keeping your weight even in your feet and your back flat with arms up.

(b) **Benefits:** Strengthens the legs and core, builds heat, opportunity to practice resilience.

4. **Wall stretches**

   a. Arms up wall (gentle option)

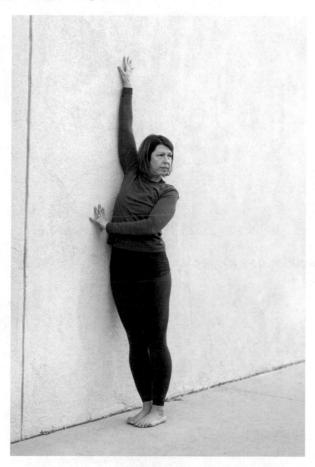

b. Arm 45° angle (moderate option)

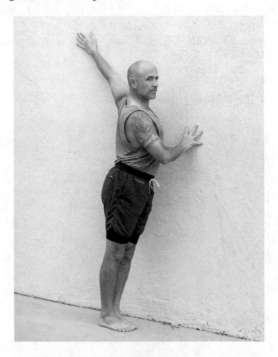

c. Arm parallel to floor (deepest option)

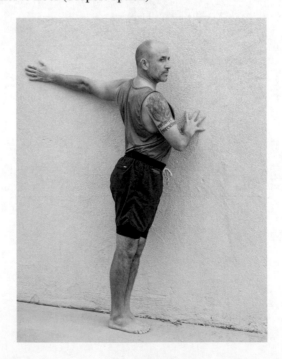

(a) **Instructions**:
    a. Gentle option: Stand with your side against the wall. Reach the arm up the wall, using the other hand on the wall for support. Slowly start to look over the shoulder opposite the wall.
    b. Moderate option: Start perpendicular to the wall and extend one arm out to a Y position (45°), using the other hand on the wall for support. Slowly start to rotate your torso away from the wall and extending arm.
    c. Deepest option: Start on the wall and extend one arm out to behind the body, using the other hand on the wall for support. Slowly start to rotate your body away from the extended arm.
(b) **Benefits:** Opens the chest and side body to relieve feelings of being hunched and tightness.

5. **Down dog on the wall**

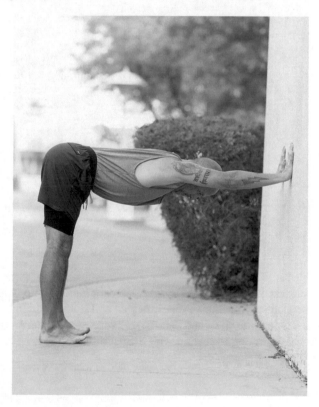

Modification – deeper

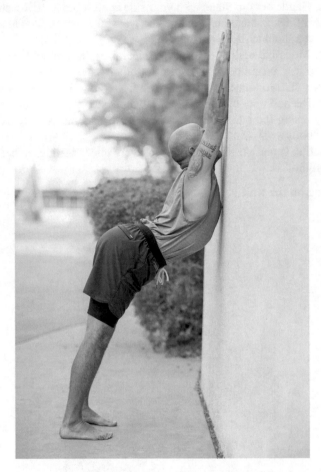

(a) **Instructions:** Start facing the wall. Place your hands at hip height and step
    back. Feet under your hips. Press into wall and squeeze thighs.
(b) **Benefits:** Opens the chest and back to relieve tension. Great modification for
    traditional down dog if dealing with a wrist or arm injury.

6. **Cat/Cow**

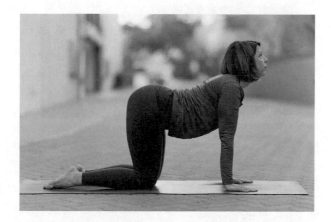

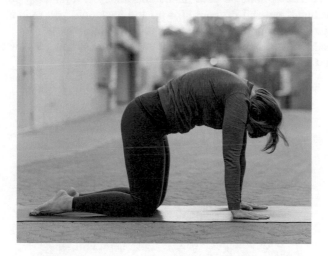

(a) **Instructions:** Start on your hands and knees in a tabletop position. As you inhale, look up, pulling chest forward, flip butt up, and lift your chest. As you exhale, round the back and shoulders as you gaze at navel.

(b) **Benefits:** Strengthens and stretches your spine. Improves focus on body and breath.

7. **Down dog**

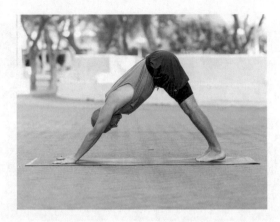

(a) **Instructions:** Start on your hands and knees in a tabletop position. Walk your hands out and lift your hips up and back until you're in an inverted V shape. Keep your back flat – it's ok to bend your knees!

(b) **Benefits:** Stretches the back you're the legs and strengthens the entire body. Good for anxiety relief. Considered a resting pose.

8. **Lying twist**

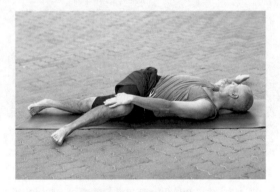

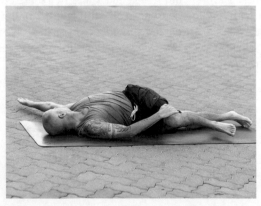

(a) **Instructions:** Lie on your back and bring one knee toward your chest. Use the opposite hand to draw the knee toward that side. Extend the other arm out in a T shape.

(b) **Benefits:** Stretches your back, hips, and glutes, and helps the body to relax.

9. **Savasana**

(a) **Instructions**: Lie on your back with legs extended (if there is any pain/discomfort in the low back, bend the knees, planting the feet on the floor. Take the feet a little bit wider than hip distance and allow the knees to fall toward each other). Close the eyes. Breathe normally (allow the ujjayi breath to fade). Rest the body completely. Allow the mind to rest. At they come into consciouness, gently let go of thoughts, feelings, and any tension that may arise. (Pause) Practice resting. Letting go. (Pause). First we let go of our physical bodies, relaxing and releasing any tension. (Pause). Then we let go of any tension in our mental and emotional bodies. We practice surrender. (Long pause). Gently begin to wiggle fingers and toes. Perhaps stretching the body as if waking from a deep sleep. Hug the knees into the chest and roll over on one side. Take a moment here. Then press up to come to sitting, opening the eyes slowly.

(b) **Benefits**: Deep rest and relaxation are underemphasized in our world. But rest is an important counterpart to movement. Practicing letting go reduces tension, improves bodily awareness, and provides us with nourishing energy.

13.4   Chapter 7 Module 3: Applications of Mindfulness

1. **Tadasana standing**

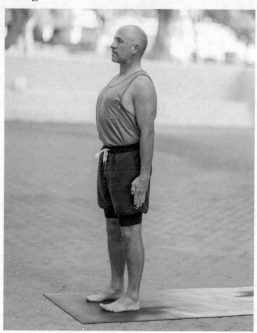

(a) **Instructions:** Stand at the front of your mat with your feet as wide as your hips. Arms can be by your sides or hand together in front of your chest.

(b) **Benefits**: Improves posture and balance.

2. **Half vinyasa**
   a. Inhale hands up

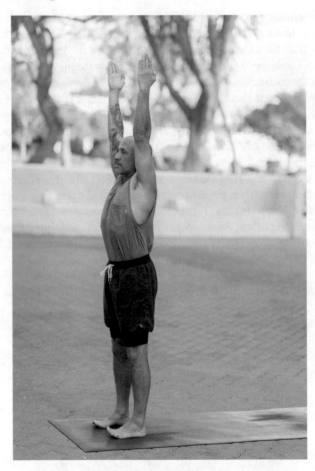

b. Forward fold exhale

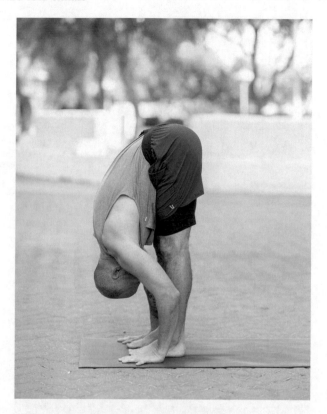

c. Inhale, head up, exhale, forward fold

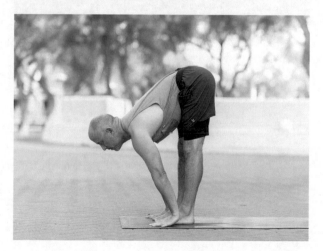

d. Inhale rise back up with arms overhead

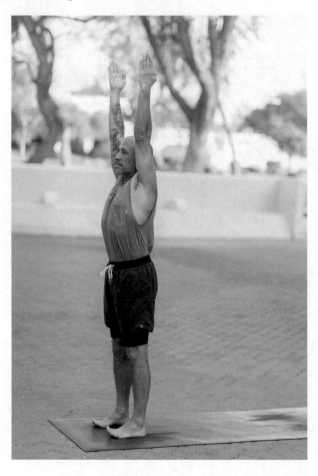

e. Exhale, tadasana standing

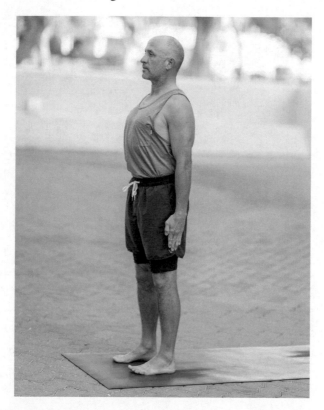

(a) **Instructions**:

a. As you inhale, lift your arms above your head keeping your ribs neutral (not lifting or splayed).

b. As you exhale, hinge at the hips as you fold forward. Place hands on ankle or floor, you can bend your knees. If your hands do touch the floor, try to flatten your hand to the floor in the same line as your toes.

c1. As you inhale, lift your head placing hands on floor or on your shins and extend your spine.

c2. As you exhale, return to your fold forward. Your hands do not need to touch the floor and you can bend your knees.

d. As you inhale, return to your first standing position, Lift your arms above your head keeping your ribs neural (not lifting or splayed).

e. As you exhale, return your arms to your sides

(b) **Benefits:** Increases blood flow, builds heat, and boosts energy.

3. **Fierce pose** (chair) hands up

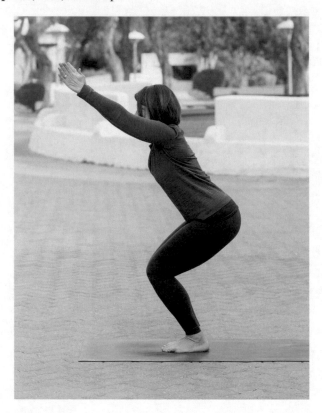

(a) **Instructions:** Bring your knees and feet together. Bend your knees and sink your hips back, keeping your weight even in your feet and your back flat with arms up.

(b) **Benefits:** Strengthens the legs and core, builds heat, opportunity to practice resilience.

4. **Cat/Cow**

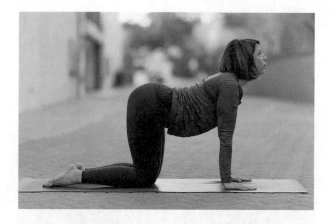

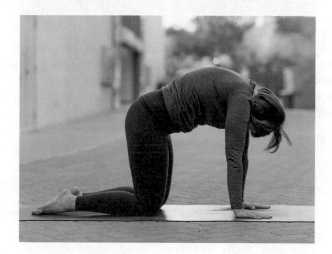

(a) **Instructions:** Start on your hands and knees in a tabletop position. As you inhale, look up, pulling chest forward, flip butt up, and lift your chest. As you exhale, round the back and shoulders as you gaze at navel.

(b) **Benefits:** Strengthens and stretches your spine. Improves focus on body and breath.

5. **Down dog**

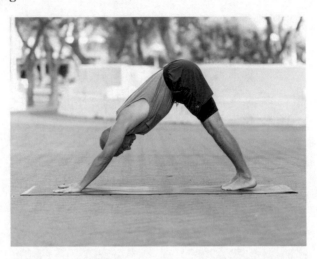

  (a) **Instructions:** Start on your hands and knees in a tabletop position. Walk
      your hands out and lift your hips up and back until you're in an inverted V
      shape. Keep your back flat – it's ok to bend your knees!
  (b) **Benefits:** Stretches the back and the legs and strengthens the entire body.
      Good for anxiety relief. Considered a resting pose.

6. **Locust pose**

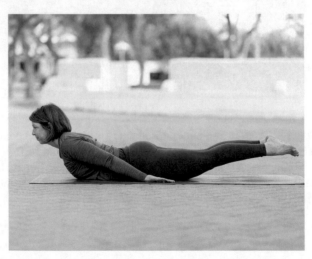

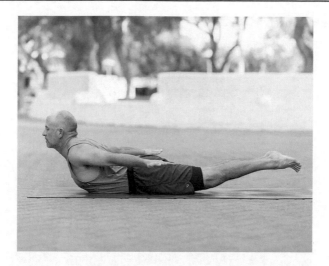

(a) **Instructions:** Start lying face down. Lift your chest, arms, and legs using the strength of your back and glutes.

(b) **Benefits:** Strengthens the back of the body and stretches the front. Helps improve posture and relieve stress.

7. **Yoga breathing or ujjayi pranayama** (no picture)

(a) **Instructions**: Find a comfortable seated position. Close your mouth and slightly constrict the back of the throat, creating an ocean-like sound. Begin with a short exhale, then inhale smoothly with the same constriction in the throat. It will sound like rolling waves of the ocean. Do this 10 times. Continue to breath in the manner during all poses.

(b) **Benefits**: Improves concentration, builds heat in the body.

8. **Tadasana** (active savasana)
   a. Arms by side

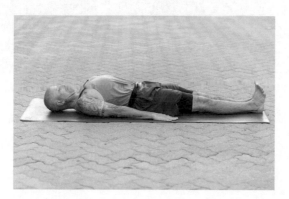

b. Arms over head

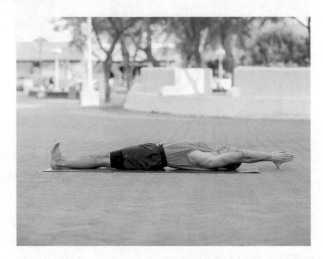

(a) **Instructions**: Lie on your mat with your feet together and actively squeeze your legs. Arms can reach either toward your feet or overhead.

(b) **Benefits**: Grounding pose that energizes the body and opens the chest.

9. **Lying twist**

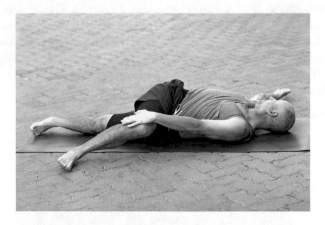

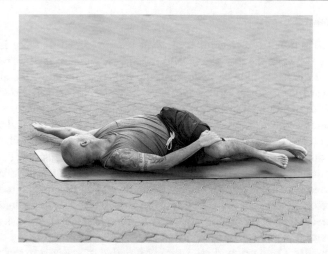

(a) **Instructions:** Lie on your back and bring one knee toward your chest. Use the opposite hand to draw the knee toward that side. Extend the other arm out in a T shape.

(b) **Benefits:** Stretches your back, hips, and glutes, and helps the body to relax.

10. **Supta Baddha Konasana**

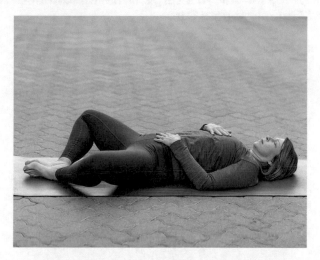

(a) **Instructions**: Lie on the floor, with the knees bent and open and the bottom of your feet together and hand on chest and belly.

(b) **Benefits**: Grounding, energizing, stress relief, stretches and opens the hips.

11. **Savasana**

(a) **Instructions**: Lie on your back with legs extended (if there is any pain/discomfort in the low back, bend the knees, planting the feet on the floor. Take the feet a little bit wider than hip distance and allow the knees to fall toward each other). Close the eyes. Breathe normally (allow the ujjayi breath to fade). Rest the body completely. Allow the mind to rest. As they come into consciouness, gently let go of thoughts, feelings, and any tension that may arise. (Pause) Practice resting. Letting go. (Pause). First we let go of our physical bodies, relaxing and releasing any tension. (Pause). Then we let go of any tension in our mental and emotional bodies. We practice surrender. (Long pause). Gently begin to wiggle fingers and toes. Perhaps stretching the body as if waking from a deep sleep. Hug the knees into the chest and roll over on one side. Take a moment here. Then press up to come to sitting, opening the eyes slowly.

(b) **Benefits**: Deep rest and relaxation are underemphasized in our world. But rest is an important counterpart to movement. Practicing letting go reduces tension, improves bodily awareness, and provides us with nourishing energy.

13.5 Chapter 8 Module 4: Interpersonal Mindfulness and Compassionate Care

1. **Tadasana standing**

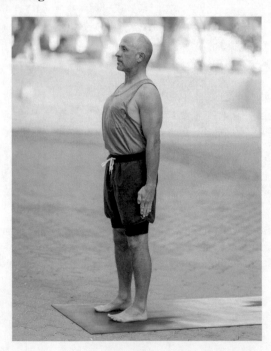

(a) **Instructions:** Stand at the front of your mat with your feet as wide as your hips. Arms can be by your sides or hand together in front of your chest.

(b) **Benefits**: Improves posture and balance.

2. **Half vinyasa**

   a. Inhale hands up

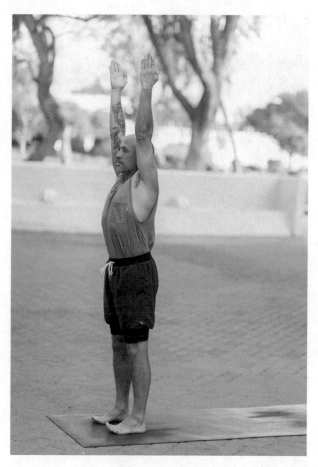

b. Forward fold exhale

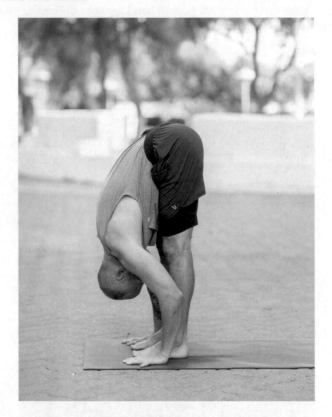

c. Inhale, head up, exhale, forward fold

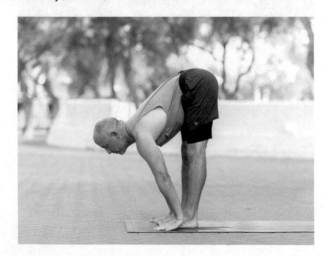

d. Inhale rise back up with arms overhead

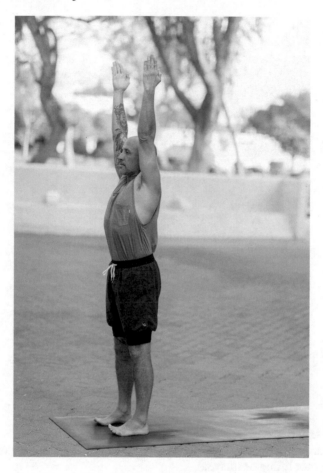

e. Exhale, tadasana standing

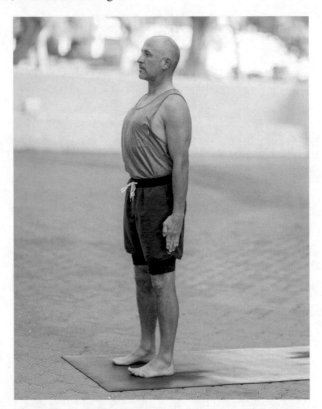

(a) **Instructions**:

a. As you inhale, lift your arms above your head keeping your ribs neutral (not lifting or splayed).

b. As you exhale, hinge at the hips as you fold forward. Place hands on ankle or floor, you can bend your knees. If your hands do touch the floor, try to flatten your hand to the floor in the same line as your toes.

c1. As you inhale, lift your head placing hands on floor or on your shins and extend your spine.

c2. As you exhale, return to your fold forward. Your hands do not need to touch the floor and you can bend your knees.

d. As you inhale, return to your first standing position, Lift your arms above your head keeping your ribs neural (not lifting or splayed).

e. As you exhale, return your arms to your sides.

(b) **Benefits:** Increases blood flow, builds heat, and boosts energy.

3. **Fierce pose** (chair) hands up

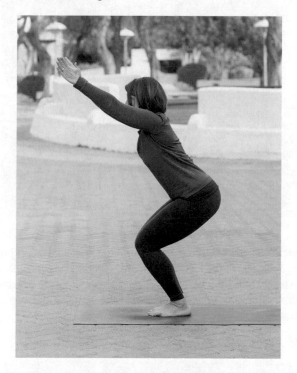

(a) **Instructions:** Bring your knees and feet together. Bend your knees and sink your hips back, keeping your weight even in your feet and your back flat with arms up.
(b) **Benefits:** Strengthens the legs and core, builds heat, opportunity to practice resilience.

4. **Cat/Cow**

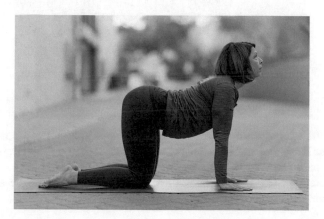

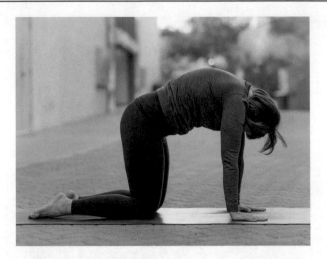

(a) **Instructions:** Start on your hands and knees in a tabletop position. As you inhale, look up, pulling chest forward, flip butt up, and lift your chest. As you exhale, round the back and shoulders as you gaze at navel.
(b) **Benefits:** Strengthens and stretches your spine. Improves focus on body and breath.

5. **Down dog**

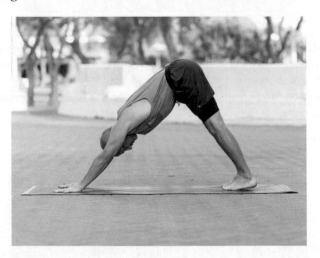

(a) **Instructions:** Start on your hands and knees in a tabletop position. Walk your hands out and lift your hips up and back until you're in an inverted V shape. Keep your back flat – it's ok to bend your knees!
(b) **Benefits:** Stretches the back of the legs and strengthens the entire body. Good for anxiety relief. Considered a resting pose.

6. **Locust pose**

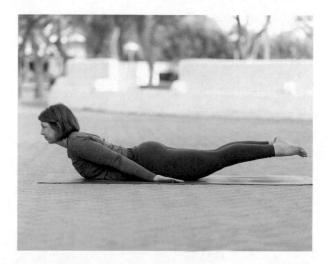

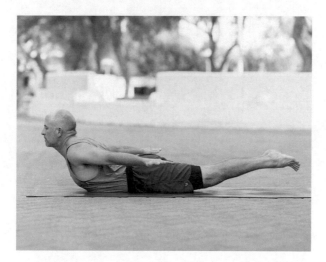

(a) **Instructions:** Start lying face down. Lift your chest, arms, and legs using the strength of your back and glutes.

(b) **Benefits:** Strengthens the back of the body and stretches the front. Helps improve posture and relieve stress.

7. **Pigeon**

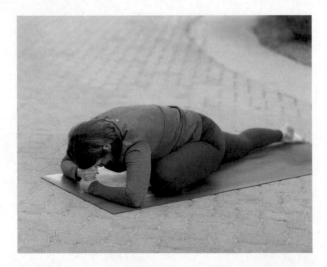

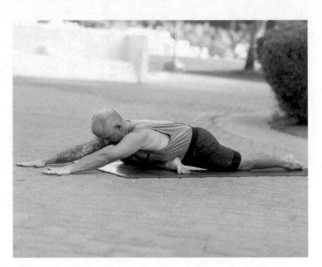

(a) **Instructions:** Bring one leg forward with your knee bent and back leg extended straight. Make sure to flex the front foot to protect your knee. You can stay upright or begin to fold forward. Put a towel or blanket under your hip.

(b) **Benefits:** Stretches the hips, which is linked to emotional release.

8. **Front and side Janu Sirsasana**

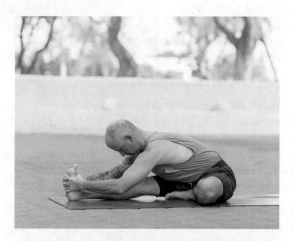

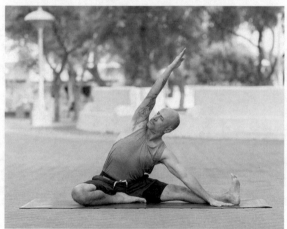

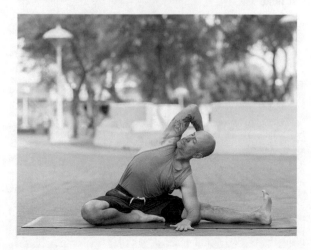

(a) **Instructions:** Start sitting and extend both legs in front of you. Bring one foot in toward your opposite thigh, keeping your knee out to the side to make a figure 4 position. Stay here or start to hinge forward, keeping your back long. Put a blanket under the knee if it is lifted.

(b) **Benefits:** Stretches the back and legs. Can help relieve anxiety and fatigue.

9. **Yoga breathing or ujjayi pranayama**

(a) **Instructions**: Find a comfortable seated position. Close your mouth and slightly constrict the back of the throat, creating an ocean-like sound. Begin with a short exhale, then inhale smoothly with the same constriction in the throat. It will sound like rolling waves of the ocean. Do this 10 times. Continue to breath in the manner during all poses.

(b) **Benefits**: Improves concentration, builds heat in the body.

10. **Tadasana** (active savasana)

a. Arms by side

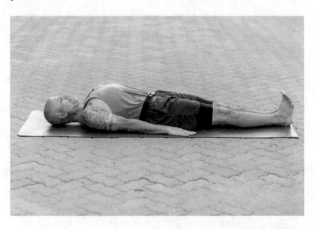

b. Arms over head

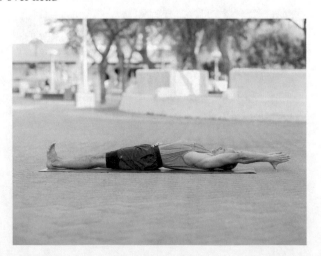

(a) **Instructions**: Lie on your mat with your feet together and actively squeeze your legs. Arms can reach either toward your feet or overhead.

(b) **Benefits**: Grounding pose that energizes the body and opens the chest.

11. **Lying twist**

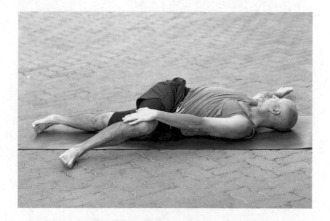

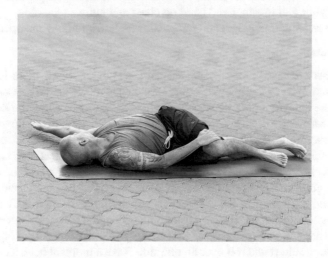

(a) **Instructions:** Lie on your back and bring one knee toward your chest. Use the opposite hand to draw the knee toward that side. Extend the other arm out in a T shape.

(b) **Benefits:** Stretches your back, hips, and glutes, and helps the body to relax.

12. **Supta Baddha Konasana**

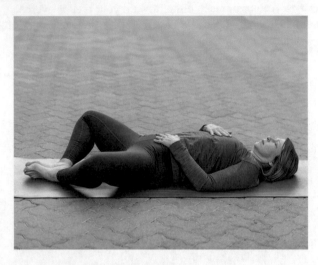

(a) **Instructions**: Lie on the floor, with the knees bent and open and the bottom of your feet together and hand on chest and belly.
(b) **Benefits**: Grounding, energizing, stress relief, stretches and opens the hips.

13. **Savasana**

(a) **Instructions**: Lie on your back with legs extended (if there is any pain/discomfort in the low back, bend the knees, planting the feet on the floor. Take the feet a little bit wider than hip distance and allow the knees to fall toward each other). Close the eyes. Breathe normally (allow the ujjayi breath to fade). Rest the body completely. Allow the mind to rest. As they come into consciousness, gently let go of thoughts, feelings, and any tension that may arise. (Pause) Practice resting. Letting go. (Pause). First we let go of our physical bodies, relaxing and releasing any tension. (Pause). Then we let go of any tension in our mental and emotional bodies. We practice surrender. (Long pause). Gently begin to wiggle fingers and toes. Perhaps stretching the body as if waking from a deep sleep. Hug the knees into the chest and roll over on one side. Take a moment here. Then press up to come to sitting, opening the eyes slowly.
(b) **Benefits**: Deep rest and relaxation are underemphasized in our world. But rest is an important counterpart to movement. Practicing letting go reduces tension, improves bodily awareness, and provides us with nourishing energy.

13.6   Chapter 10 Module 6: Mindful Compassion in the Presence of Suffering

1. **Tadasana standing**

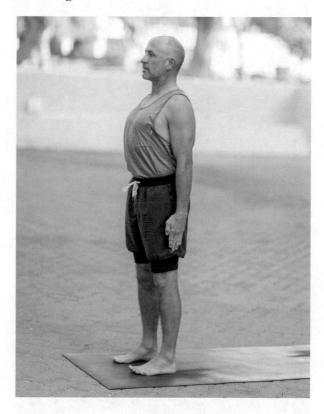

(a) **Instructions:** Stand at the front of your mat with your feet as wide as your hips. Arms can be by your sides or hand together in front of your chest.
(b) **Benefits**: Improves posture and balance.

2. **Half vinyasa**
   a. Inhale hands up

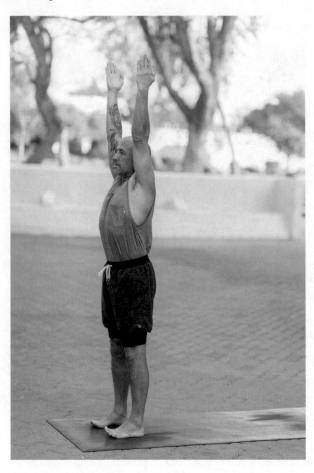

b. Forward fold exhale

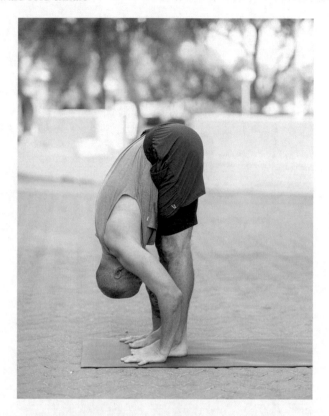

c. Inhale, head up, exhale, forward fold

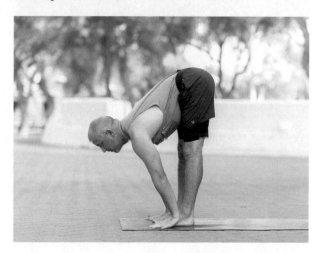

d. Inhale rise back up with arms overhead

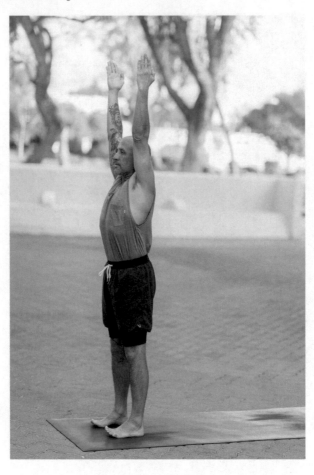

e. Exhale, tadasana standing

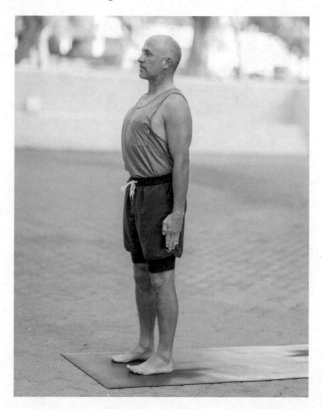

(a) **Instructions**:

    a. As you inhale, lift your arms above your head keeping your ribs neutral (not lifting or splayed).

    b. As you exhale, hinge at the hips as you fold forward. Place hands on ankle or floor, you can bend your knees. If your hands do touch the floor, try to flatten your hand to the floor in the same line as your toes.

    c1. As you inhale, lift your head placing hands on floor or on your shins and extend your spine.

    c2. As you exhale, return to your fold forward. Your hands do not need to touch the floor and you can bend your knees.

    d. As you inhale, return to your first standing position, Lift your arms above your head keeping your ribs neural (not lifting or splayed).

    e. As you exhale, return your arms to your sides

(b) **Benefits:** Increases blood flow, builds heat, and boosts energy.

3. **Fierce pose** (chair) hands up

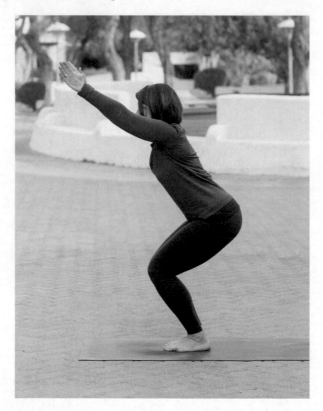

(a) **Instructions:** Bring your knees and feet together. Bend your knees and sink your hips back, keeping your weight even in your feet and your back flat with arms up.

(b) **Benefits:** Strengthens the legs and core, builds heat, opportunity to practice resilience.

4. **Tree pose**

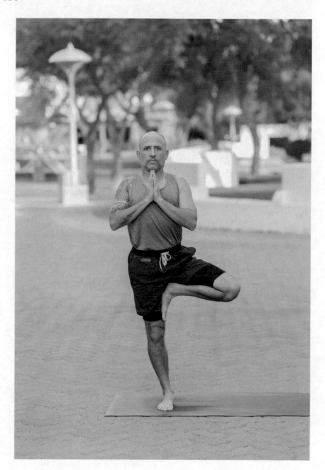

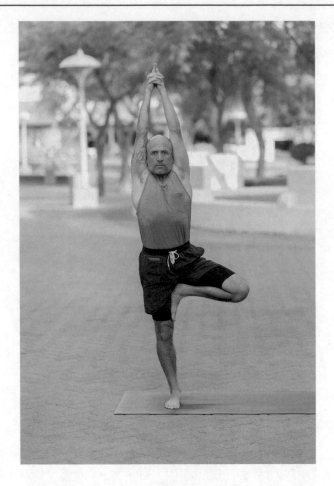

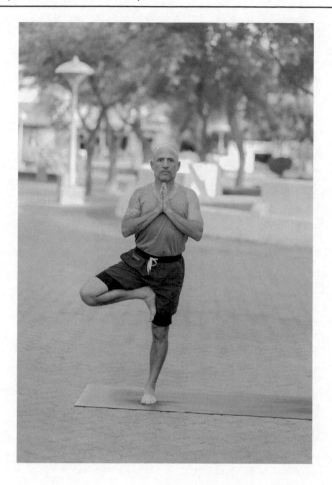

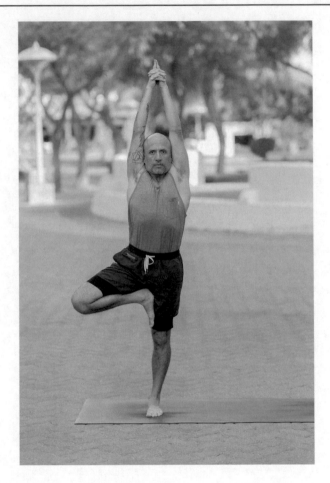

(a) **Instructions:** Start standing and shift your weight over to one leg. Bend the opposite knee, bringing it out to the side. Bring your foot to either your ankle, calf, or thigh, but avoid the knee. Press heel into thigh.

(b) **Benefits:** Improves balance and strengthens leg and core muscles. Also improves focus.

5. **Warrior 2 modified** – both sides

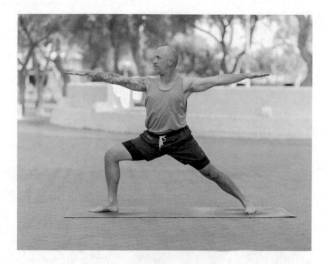

(right side)

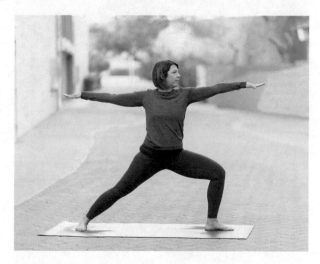

(left side)

(a) **Instructions:** Start in a wide stance (approx. 4 ft) facing the long edge of your mat. Turn your front toes 90° so that the front heel lines up with the back arch. Bend into the front knee (90°) and raise the arms to a T position, gazing over the front fingers.

(b) **Benefits:** Strengthens core and leg muscles, builds heat in the body, and improves concentration and stamina.

6. **Side angle modified** – both sides

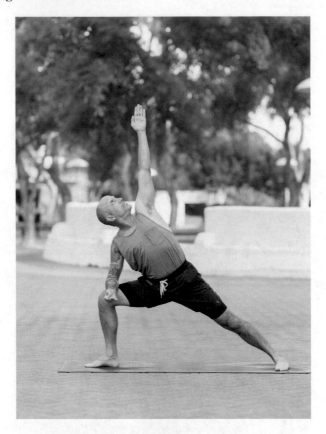

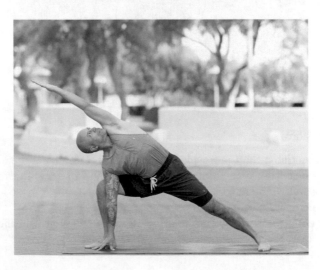

(right side)

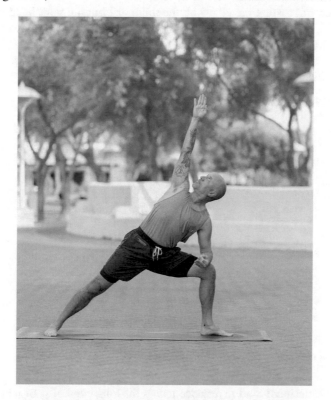

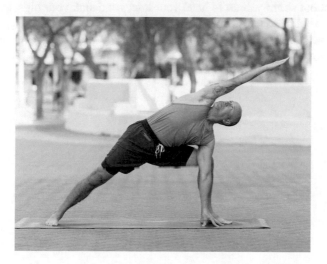

(left side)

(a) **Instructions:** from Warrior 2, reach the front arm out and start to hinge forward, resting the elbow on the thigh or bringing your hand to the floor. Keep your core engaged. The other arm can either extend upward or beside the ear.

(b) **Benefits:** Strengthens core and leg muscles, stretches the side of the body, builds heat, and improves concentration and stamina.

7. **Goddess**

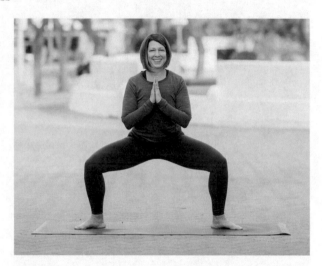

(a) **Instructions:** Start in a stance facing the long edge of your mat. Turn your feet out slightly. Start to bend your knees and sink your hips, keeping your knees aligned with your toes.

(b) **Benefits:** Strengthens core, legs, and pelvic floor. Improves stamina and focus, opens the hips.

8. **Runner and twist**

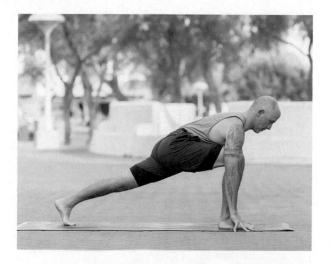

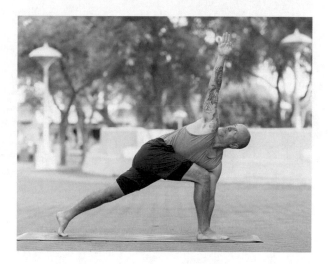

(right side)

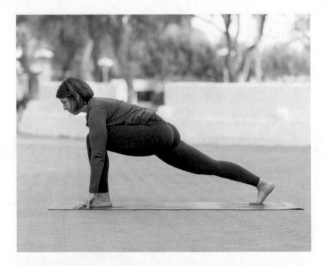

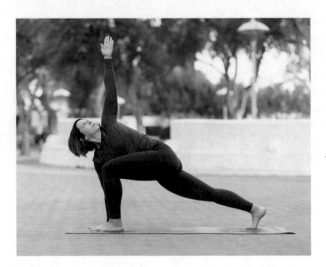

(left side)

(a) **Instructions:** (1) Step one foot to opposite thumb, keeping your chest up and core lifted. You can place your hands on two blocks or books. (2) Plant the palm of your hand opposite the forward leg, close to the foot, and raise the other hand on the same side.

(b) **Benefits:** Stretches the legs and opens tight hips. Improves thoracic spine mobility.

9. **Supta Baddha Konasana**

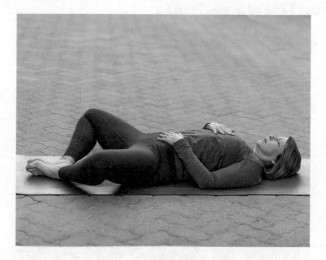

(a) **Instructions**: Lie on the floor, with the knees bent and open and the bottom of your feet together and hand on chest and belly.

(b) **Benefits**: Grounding, energizing, stress relief, stretches and opens the hips.

10. **Savasana**

(a) **Instructions**: Lie on your back with legs extended (if there is any pain/discomfort in the low back, bend the knees, planting the feet on the floor. Take the feet a little bit wider than hip distance and allow the knees to fall toward each other). Close the eyes. Breathe normally (allow the ujjayi breath to fade). Rest the body completely. Allow the mind to rest. As they come into consciousness, gently let go of thoughts, feelings, and any tension that may arise. (Pause) Practice resting. Letting go. (Pause). First we let go of our physical bodies, relaxing and releasing any tension. (Pause). Then we let go of any tension in our mental and emotional bodies. We practice surrender. (Long pause). Gently begin to wiggle fingers and toes. Perhaps stretching the body as if waking from a deep sleep. Hug the knees into the chest and roll over on one side. Take a moment here. Then press up to come to sitting, opening the eyes slowly.

(b) **Benefits**: Deep rest and relaxation are underemphasized in our world. But rest is an important counterpart to movement. Practicing letting go reduces tension, improves bodily awareness, and provides us with nourishing energy.

13.7 Chapter 11 Module 7: Mindfulness and Compassion in the Face of Imperfection

In between each pose, rest as needed in child's pose.

1. **Tadasana standing**

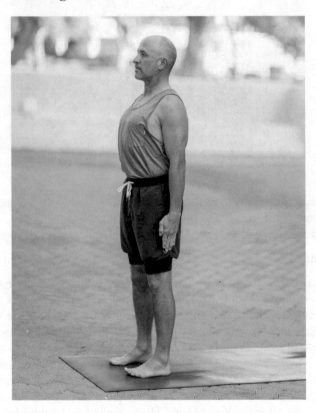

   (a) **Instructions:** Stand at the front of your mat with your feet as wide as your hips. Arms can be by your sides or hand together in front of your chest.
   (b) **Benefits**: Improves posture and balance.

2. **Half vinyasa**
   a. Inhale hands up

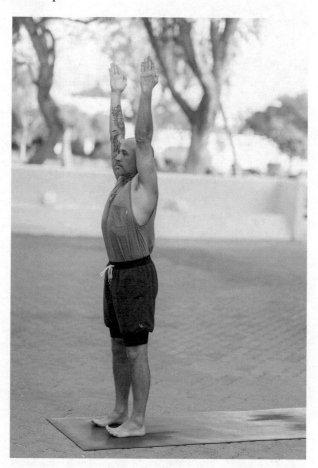

b. Forward fold exhale

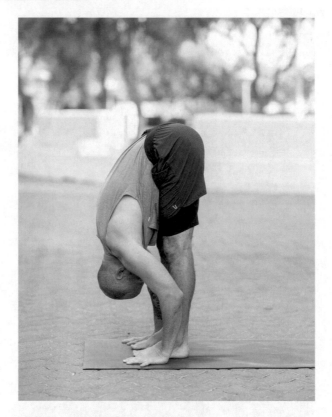

c. Inhale, head up, exhale, forward fold

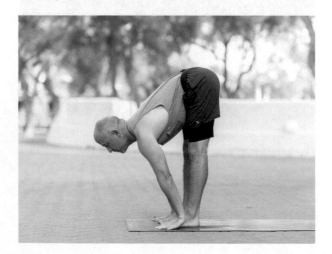

d. Inhale rise back up with arms overhead

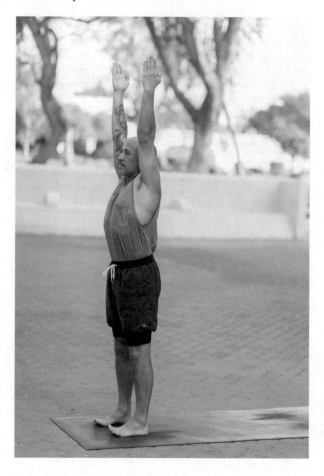

e. Exhale, tadasana standing

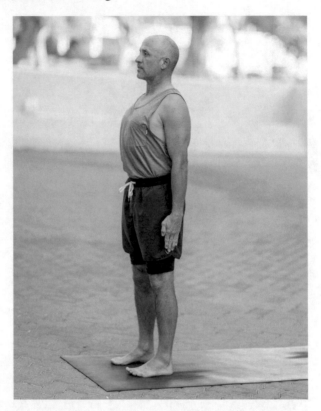

(a) **Instructions:**

   a. As you inhale, lift your arms above your head keeping your ribs neutral (not lifting or splayed).

   b. As you exhale, hinge at the hips as you fold forward. Place hands on ankle or floor, you can bend your knees. If your hands do touch the floor, try to flatten your hand to the floor in the same line as your toes.

   c1. As you inhale, lift your head placing hands on floor or on your shins and extend your spine.

   c2. As you exhale, return to your fold forward. Your hands do not need to touch the floor and you can bend your knees.

   d. As you inhale, return to your first standing position, Lift your arms above your head keeping your ribs neural (not lifting or splayed).

   e. As you exhale, return your arms to your sides

(b) **Benefits:** Increases blood flow, builds heat, and boosts energy.

3. **Fierce pose** (chair) hands up

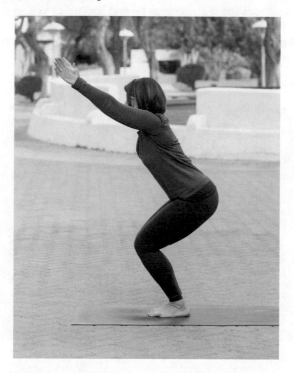

   (a) **Instructions:** Bring your knees and feet together. Bend your knees and sink your hips back, keeping your weight even in your feet and your back flat with arms up.

   (b) **Benefits:** Strengthens the legs and core, builds heat, opportunity to practice resilience.

4. **Down dog**

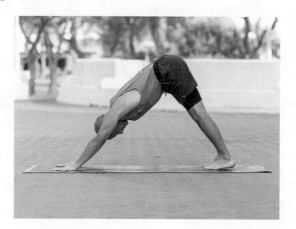

(a) **Instructions:** Start on your hands and knees in a tabletop position. Walk your hands out and lift your hips up and back until you're in an inverted V shape. Keep your back flat – it's ok to bend your knees!

(b) **Benefits:** Stretches the back and the legs and strengthens the entire body. Good for anxiety relief. Considered a resting pose.

5. **Locust pose**

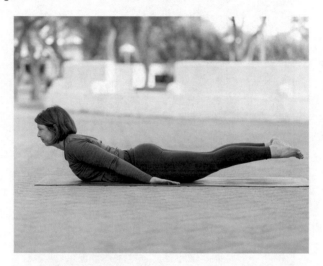

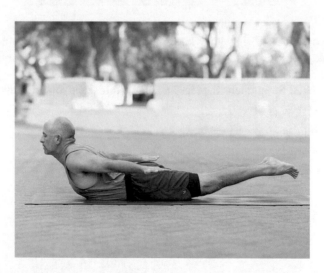

(a) **Instructions:** Start lying face down. Lift your chest, arms, and legs using the strength of your back and glutes.

(b) **Benefits:** Strengthens the back of the body and stretches the front. Helps improve posture and relieve stress.

6. **Bow pose**

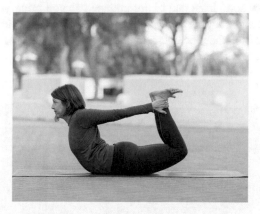

(a) **Instructions:** Start lying face down. Lift your chest, arms, and legs using the strength of your back and glutes. Begin to bend your knees and reach your arms back to catch your ankles on the outside.

(b) **Benefits:** Strengthens the back of the body and stretches the front, with a deeper stretch in the chest and shoulders. Helps improve posture and relieve stress.

7. **Camel**

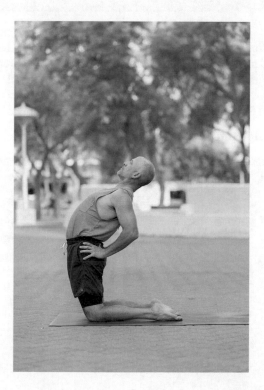

(a) **Instructions:** Begin kneeling with your toes either tucked or untucked. Keep your core, legs, and glutes engaged as you bring your hands to your low back and lift your chest. Stay here for several breaths.

(b) **Benefits:** Stretches the chest, abdomen, and quadriceps, while strengthening the back of the body. Opens the heart.

8. **Pigeon**

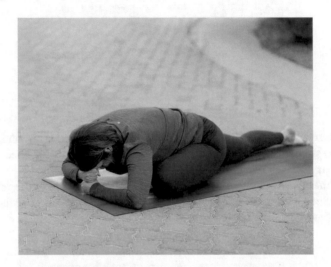

(a) **Instructions:** Bring one leg forward with your knee bent and back leg extended straight. Make sure to flex the front foot to protect your knee. You can stay upright or begin to fold forward. Put a towel or blanket under your hip.

(b) **Benefits:** Stretches the hips, which is linked to emotional release.

9. **Front and side Janu Sirsasana**

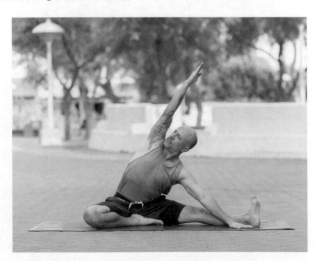

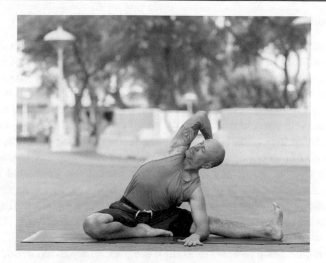

(a) **Instructions:** Start sitting and extend both legs in front of you. Bring one foot in toward your opposite thigh, keeping your knee out to the side to make a figure 4 position. Stay here or start to hinge forward, keeping your back long. Put a blanket under the knee if it is lifted.

(b) **Benefits:** Stretches the back and legs. Can help relieve anxiety and fatigue.

10. **Supta Baddha Konasana**

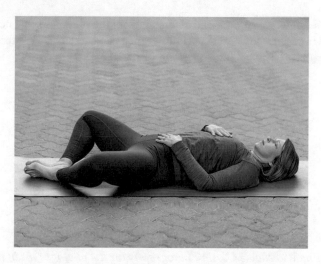

(a) **Instructions**: Lie on the floor, with the knees bent and open and the bottom of your feet together and hand on chest and belly.

(b) **Benefits**: Grounding, energizing, stress relief, stretches and opens the hips.

11. **Savasana**

(a) **Instructions**: Lie on your back with legs extended (if there is any pain/discomfort in the low back, bend the knees, planting the feet on the floor. Take the feet a little bit wider than hip distance and allow the knees to fall toward each other). Close the eyes. Breathe normally (allow the ujjayi breath to fade). Rest the body completely. Allow the mind to rest. As they come into consciousness, gently let go of thoughts, feelings, and any tension that may arise. (Pause) Practice resting. Letting go. (Pause). First we let go of our physical bodies, relaxing and releasing any tension. (Pause). Then we let go of any tension in our mental and emotional bodies. We practice surrender. (Long pause). Gently begin to wiggle fingers and toes. Perhaps stretching the body as if waking from a deep sleep. Hug the knees into the chest and roll over on one side. Take a moment here. Then press up to come to sitting, opening the eyes slowly.

(b) **Benefits**: Deep rest and relaxation are underemphasized in our world. But rest is an important counterpart to movement. Practicing letting go reduces tension, improves bodily awareness, and provides us with nourishing energy.

13.8   Chapter 12 Module 8: Finding Balance Through Mindful Living

For the last module, we recommend choosing from the previous sequences or creating your own based on the students' preferences and interest. Poll the class! Are there any requests? Make it fun and group centered.

With gratitude to Nicole Curtin Photography for the photographs in this chapter.

Printed in the United States
by Baker & Taylor Publisher Services